Mayo Clinic on Crohn's Disease & Ulcerative Colitis

**Strategies to manage IBD
and take charge of your life**

Francis A. Farraye, M.D., M.Sc. | **Sunanda V. Kane, M.D., M.S.P.H.**

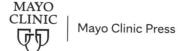 Mayo Clinic Press

MAYO CLINIC PRESS

Medical Editors | Francis A. Farraye, M.D., M.Sc., Sunanda V. Kane, M.D., M.S.P.H.
Publisher | Daniel J. Harke
Editor in Chief | Nina E. Wiener
Senior Editor | Karen R. Wallevand
Art Director | Stewart J. Koski
Production Design | Gunnar T. Soroos
Contributor | Jaclyn R. Elkins, M.S., R.D.N.
Image Credits | All photographs and illustrations are copyright of Mayo Foundation for Medical Education and Research (MFMER)

Additional contributions from Marci Reiss, L.C.S.W., Orvos Communications, Kirkus Reviews and Rath Indexing

To stay informed about Mayo Clinic Press, please subscribe to our free e-newsletter at MCPress.MayoClinic.org or follow us on social media.

Published by Mayo Clinic Press

The information in this book is true and complete to the best of our knowledge. This book is intended only as an informative guide for those wishing to learn more about health issues. It is not intended to replace, countermand or conflict with advice given to you by your own physician. The ultimate decision concerning your care should be made between you and your doctor. Information in this book is offered with no guarantees. The authors and publisher disclaim all liability in connection with the use of this book.

For bulk sales to employers, member groups and health-related companies, contact Mayo Clinic, 200 First St. SW, Rochester, MN 55905, or email SpecialSalesMayoBooks@mayo.edu.

ISBN 978-1-945564-08-6
Library of Congress Control Number: 2022931297

Printed in the United States of America

When you purchase Mayo Clinic newsletters and books, proceeds are used to further medical education and research at Mayo Clinic. You not only get answers to your questions on health, you become part of the solution.

I dedicate this book to my supportive and loving family: my wife, Renee M. Remily, M.D., my children, Jennifer Farraye, M.S.N., N.P., and Alexis Farraye; and to my parents, who taught me that perseverance and commitment can result in great accomplishments. I thank my patients and their families for their confidence in allowing me to care for them.

Francis Farraye

This book is dedicated to my father, who pushed me incessantly because he knew I could accomplish great things if I just put my mind to it. To Stephen Hanauer, M.D., the best role model a young physician could ever have. He taught me the art of caring for patients, and I will always be indebted to him. And to my husband, who was so exquisitely patient, caring and supportive while I spent even less time with him than usual to write this book.

Sunanda Kane

Acknowledgments

Writing this book was a true labor of love. It embodies all the things that we'd want to teach you if you were a patient of ours. We cover many topics; however, because the inflammatory bowel disease (IBD) field is changing quickly, it's impossible to touch on everything. Also, IBD is a personal disease: How it affects you and what you need to do to live with it successfully are unique to you. To get the most out of this book, read it through the lens of your own challenges and goals.

As we discuss in detail the difficulties of living with IBD, our intent is not to become the voice of gloom and doom. Just the opposite. We fully believe that the more you understand your disease and possible treatment options, the better you'll be able to live fully. The majority of our patients lead productive, happy and well-adjusted lives. In addition, the prognosis for both ulcerative colitis and Crohn's disease has become much brighter in recent decades. Newer therapies that allow the intestines to heal and surgery that spares the bowel and provides more cosmetically appealing outcomes are emerging. We feel very fortunate to be part of a field that's significantly improving people's lives.

Nutrition is an important concern for most people with IBD and the topic for which we get the most questions. We turned to Jaclyn Elkins, M.S., R.D.N., C.N.S.C., an expert in IBD nutritional management and advanced nutrition support, for major contributions to Chapter 10. Jaclyn is a clinical dietitian at Mayo Clinic, Jacksonville, Fla., and an instructor in nutrition at Mayo Clinic College of Medicine and Science.

For information on children and adolescents, we sought input and counsel from Marci Reiss, L.C.S.W., a dedicated social worker who assists families of children with IBD struggling to find normalcy in their lives. In Chapter 13, she kindly shares some sage advice for parents. Marci is also the president of the IBD Support Foundation, a worthy organization that provides support programs for patients and families with ulcerative colitis and Crohn's disease.

The information in this book is based on clinical research, controlled trials, personal experiences and communications with trusted colleagues. We also asked many of our patients with IBD what they'd like to see in a book, and we listened. *Mayo Clinic on Crohn's Disease and Ulcerative Colitis* is for everyone affected by the disease, including many of you we'll never meet but want to help.

Francis A. Farraye, M.D., M.Sc.
Sunanda V. Kane, M.D., M.S.P.H.

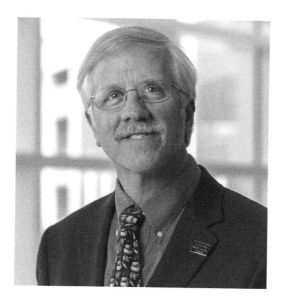

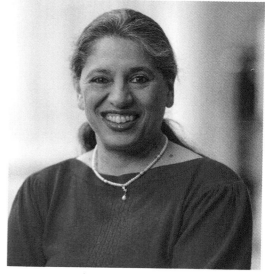

Francis A. Farraye, M.D., M.Sc., is the director of the Inflammatory Bowel Disease Center at Mayo Clinic, Jacksonville, Fla., and a professor of medicine at Mayo Clinic College of Medicine and Science. A gastroenterologist and clinical investigator, he has been practicing medicine for 33 years. Dr. Farraye is a frequent speaker on the diagnosis and management of IBD and has authored or coauthored more than 450 scientific manuscripts, chapters, reviews and abstracts. He is editor in chief of *IBD Journal Scan* published weekly by the American Society of Gastrointestinal Endoscopy. He coedited the publications *Curbside Consultation in Inflammatory Bowel Disease* and *GI Emergencies*. The New England Crohn's & Colitis Foundation named him their humanitarian of the year (2003) and gave him their lifetime achievement award (2020). In 2009, he received the William Carey Award from the American College of Gastroenterology for service to the college. Dr. Farraye lives in Jacksonville, Fla.

Sunanda V. Kane, M.D., M.S.P.H., is a professor of medicine at Mayo Clinic College of Medicine and Science and assistant chair for patient experience within the division of Gastroenterology and Hepatology, Mayo Clinic, Rochester, Minn. She also serves as chair of Mayo Clinic Quality Academy's fellow subcommittee. Dr. Kane, a gastroenterologist and clinical investigator, has been practicing medicine for 22 years. She served as president of the American College of Gastroenterology from 2018 to 2019, chaired the National Patient Education Committee for the Crohn's & Colitis Foundation and recently completed a five-year term on the Gastroenterology Specialty Council for the American Board of Internal Medicine. Dr. Kane authored the book *IBD Self-Management*, published by the American Gastroenterological Association. She has written more than 200 chapters, articles and reviews, and she serves in other editorial roles. Dr. Kane lives in Rochester, Minn.

Foreword

Whether you're newly diagnosed with Crohn's disease or ulcerative colitis or you've been living with inflammatory bowel disease (IBD) for many years, having accurate, unbiased and credible information is essential to your health. Finding a trusted resource on IBD can be a daunting task. It's easy to feel overwhelmed and confused by the sea of information, whether exploring the disease on the internet or reviewing the vast array of scientific research, books and personal stories.

The Crohn's & Colitis Foundation supports millions of patients and caregivers searching for information on managing IBD. Informational needs range from understanding Crohn's disease and ulcerative colitis, available treatment options and therapies on the horizon, diet and nutrition guidance, and emotional and mental support resources. It's the Foundation's priority to connect people with accurate information, equipping them with the knowledge and tools they need to work with their health care team to improve their quality of life and manage their disease toward remission.

The Crohn's & Colitis Foundation is enthusiastic about adding *Mayo Clinic on Crohn's Disease and Ulcerative Colitis*, authored by Dr. Francis Farraye and Dr. Sunanda Kane, to our IBD Help Center resources.

This valuable guide can be shared with anyone living with IBD and with family and friends supporting someone with IBD. The chapters are easy to read and written in a supportive voice. The book is filled with patient stories, bringing to life the diverse experiences of living with Crohn's disease and ulcerative colitis.

Drs. Francis Farraye and Sunanda Kane are dedicated volunteers supporting the IBD community. They've shared their time, wisdom and expertise as members of the Crohn's & Colitis Foundation National Scientific Advisory Committee. They've also participated in educational and advocacy programs to help ensure access to treatments, procedures and providers through our state and federal advocacy programs.

It's been my pleasure to work with Drs. Farraye and Kane for more than a decade.

Until there's a cure for Crohn's disease and ulcerative colitis, there will continue to be a vital need for comprehensive, evidence-based resources to support all individuals living with or affected by IBD.

Laura D. Wingate
Executive Vice President, Education, Support & Advocacy Crohn's & Colitis Foundation

Contents

4   Acknowledgments

6   Foreword

12   CHAPTER 1
WHY IBD? WHY ME?

Understanding the gastrointestinal tract
Inflammatory bowel disease defined
Were you misdiagnosed?
Clues as to a cause
Dealing with your feelings
Telling others

26   CHAPTER 2
UNDERSTANDING ULCERATIVE COLITIS

Symptoms of ulcerative colitis
Diagnosing ulcerative colitis
Managing ulcerative colitis

37   CHAPTER 3
UNDERSTANDING CROHN'S DISEASE

Types of Crohn's disease
Symptoms of Crohn's disease
Diagnosing Crohn's disease
Managing Crohn's disease

46   CHAPTER 4
OTHER TYPES OF IBD

Indeterminate colitis
Microscopic or lymphocytic colitis
Collagenous colitis

50   CHAPTER 5
SELF-MANAGEMENT: IT'S YOUR IBD

Immediate plan
Short-term plan
Long-term plan
Health care team
Getting the most from your visits

60   CHAPTER 6
MEDICATIONS FOR IBD

Anti-inflammatory medications
Immunomodulators
Biologics
Small molecules
Antibiotics
Medications for specific symptoms
Future treatments
Clinical trials
Staying on your medication
Complementary therapies

92 **CHAPTER 7**
        IBD AFFECTS MORE THAN YOUR GUT

Eyes
Liver
Kidneys
Bones
Joints
Hair, teeth and nails
Skin

100 **CHAPTER 8**
         THE IBD-CANCER CONNECTION

Cancer risk
Preventing colorectal cancer
Dealing with dysplasia
Medications to prevent colorectal cancer
Other types of cancer

107 **CHAPTER 9**
         WHEN YOU NEED SURGERY

Types of surgery
Surgery for ulcerative colitis
Surgery for Crohn's disease
Postoperative complications
Stomas

124 **CHAPTER 10**
         THE FOOD FIGHT: WHAT CAN YOU EAT?

A nutritional challenge
Nutrition 101: What every body needs
Your individual nutrition needs
Fiber and residue
Lactose intolerance
Calcium: A special problem
Trigger foods
Reactions to gluten and more
Your need for glutamine
Malnutrition in IBD

When you can't eat food
Diets specifically for IBD
General guidelines for healthy eating

153   CHAPTER 11
TAKING CHARGE OF YOUR LIFESTYLE

Pain
Stress
Anxiety and depression
Sleep and fatigue
Tobacco use
Physical activity
Travel
Work

160   CHAPTER 12
SEX, FERTILITY AND PREGNANCY

Men
Women
Fertility and pregnancy

170   CHAPTER 13
GROWING UP WITH IBD

Growth and development
Differences in children and teens
Treating IBD in children and teens
Monitoring IBD in children and teens
Staying on medication
Fitting in with IBD
Advice on common parental issues

183   Additional resources
184   Index

1

Why IBD? Why me?

Life is hard for Joanna. She needs to know where the nearest bathroom is at all times and lives in constant fear that she'll have an accident. Her health has put a big dent in her social life, and she often turns down invitations to events and gatherings. Joanna's joints hurt, and she's much more fatigued than she thinks a 27-year-old should be.

Does this sound like you? We hope not, but if you have inflammatory bowel disease (IBD), this is how you may feel when your disease is active or under-treated. IBD is an umbrella term used to describe disorders that involve chronic inflammation of the digestive tract, including Crohn's disease and ulcerative colitis. It's a lifelong condition, but it doesn't have to be an "illness."

What's sad about Joanna is that she's become angry, complacent and disillusioned about her situation. She dwells on

the idea that she can't be helped, and once this happens, improvement is almost impossible. Joanna repeatedly refuses referrals to a medical center that specializes in treating IBD, despite the urging of her doctors. Instead, she puts her faith in individuals she's always seen for her health and expects them to know everything. Joanna stops her medicines without telling anyone, for one reason or another. Rather than keeping her scheduled appointments, she relies on the local hospital emergency room when she finds herself in need of urgent care. She reads

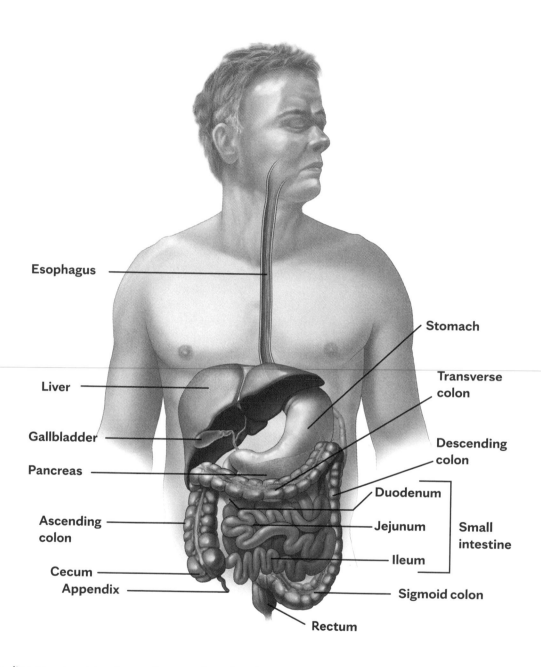

Esophagus

Stomach

Liver

Transverse colon

Gallbladder

Descending colon

Pancreas

Duodenum

Ascending colon

Jejunum

Small intestine

Cecum

Ileum

Appendix

Sigmoid colon

Rectum

The digestive tract begins at the mouth and ends at the rectum and includes several internal organs. Food moves through your body along the digestive tract.

internet sites that scare her more than educate her and takes advice from well-meaning but uninformed friends, neighbors and coworkers. She won't take the vitamins her doctors suggest, even though she knows she's iron deficient. She often asks, "Why me?"

It's obvious to everyone but Joanna that she isn't willing to help herself. Doctors understand that some people can't be helped, but they also are aware that some people *won't* be helped. Although there's no cure for IBD, there are ways to treat it, which are improving every day. But doctors can only do so much.

The truth is, how you fare with IBD is partially your choice. You need to believe that there's a path to making peace and finding health. You can find your own way by taking control of your body and your disease and learning all that you can about responsible ways to help yourself. This book offers proven and reliable information on how to live your best life. Having met and cared for thousands of people facing IBD, we're convinced that you have the ability to succeed at living with and managing your IBD.

UNDERSTANDING THE GASTROINTESTINAL TRACT

To manage your IBD, it's important to understand how the gastrointestinal (GI) tract works. It starts in the mouth and ends at the anus and includes several internal organs, including the esophagus, stomach, small intestine, colon and rectum. The small intestine is divided into three sections — the duodenum, jejunum and ileum. The terminal ileum comprises the last few inches of the ileum.

The colon is also referred to as the large intestine or bowel. It's divided into three basic parts: the right side (cecum and ascending colon), left side (descending colon and sigmoid colon) and rectum. Although it's physically attached to the colon, the rectum is supplied by a different network of nerves and blood vessels than the rest of the colon, so it's considered its own section. The transverse colon, located on top, bridges the right and left sides and is divided between the two. The appendix hangs from the cecum, the beginning of the large intestine.

The colon is composed of multiple layers. The innermost layer of cells, called the mucosa, absorbs water from stool. This is the main function of the colon: to absorb water from waste material passed on from the small intestine after digestion and to package it for removal from the body. The mucosa, which can be seen with a medical device called an endoscope, is the part of the colon that's sampled during a biopsy. The other layers, moving from the inside to the outside, are connective tissue, muscle and an outer lining that contains nerve cells.

In addition to these layers, there are glands in the rectum and colon that produce mucus. Mucus helps lubricate stool so that it slides out more readily when you're having a bowel movement. Normally, mucus stays within the rectum and you don't see it. It gets reabsorbed and new mucus is produced. When there's inflammation or irritation in the colon, these glands become more active and additional mucus is produced. In the case of diarrhea, mucus may come out with the stool rather than staying within the rectum. Mucus in the stool is often a sign of inflammation, but it may occur with other conditions, such as irritable bowel syndrome (see page 17).

More on inflammation

Inflammation is the body's reaction to anything foreign. It's a natural process that's essential for health. "Foreign" can be practically anything — from a splinter in your finger to the poison in a bee sting to the bacteria in tainted tuna salad. The natural reaction of your body to this foreign invader is to attack it in an effort to get rid of it, either by engulfing and digesting it or by destroying it. We experience inflammation as swelling, redness, warmth and pain, all caused by proteins that are produced during the attack-and-destroy process.

Sometimes the body is tricked into thinking that some portion or product of itself is foreign, causing the body to attack itself. This is what's called an autoimmune reaction. There are many examples of autoimmune diseases, such as lupus, type 1 diabetes, rheumatoid arthritis and inflammatory bowel disease.

INFLAMMATORY BOWEL DISEASE DEFINED

IBD is characteristically a lifelong (chronic) condition in which the lining of the gastrointestinal tract becomes inflamed for no apparent reason. The inflammation might be located in just one part of the digestive tract, for example, in the large intestine (colon), but it can appear anywhere along the digestive tract, from the mouth to the anus.

IBD occurs in different forms. There are two major types and two less common types. Ulcerative colitis, discussed in Chapter 2, and Crohn's disease, discussed in Chapter 3, are the most common and most recognizable forms. Chapter 4 looks at other less common types of IBD.

More than 1.6 million Americans have IBD, split about equally between Crohn's disease and ulcerative colitis. However,

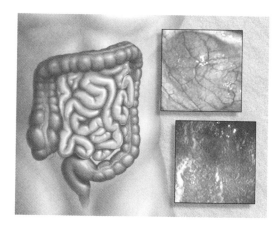

The images on the right show the innermost lining of the large intestine. The top image depicts a healthy large intestine. The bottom image shows inflammation characteristic of IBD.

Miriam, a 72-year-old woman with bad arthritis of the knees, was referred for "unresolving colitis." She takes ibuprofen on a regular basis for her knee pain and developed blood in her stools and was worried that she had colon cancer. An exam of her lower digestive tract revealed inflammation of Miriam's colon, and samples from the lining of her colon (biopsies) also seemed to indicate nonspecific inflammation. Believing that Miriam had ulcerative colitis, her doctor started her on specific medications, but she continued to bleed. Despite even stronger medications, her symptoms continued. That's when Miriam was referred to a specialty center for a second opinion. Her biopsies were carefully reviewed under a microscope. It turned out that Miriam had acute, not chronic, inflammation, more consistent with damage from taking ibuprofen rather than a chronic condition like ulcerative colitis. She discontinued the ulcerative colitis medications and received information on physical therapy to manage her knee pain rather than high doses of ibuprofen. After a couple of weeks off ibuprofen, Miriam's rectal bleeding stopped, and a follow-up exam confirmed resolution of the inflammation.

this balance is likely to change. The number of new cases of Crohn's disease is on the rise, although the reason behind this trend isn't entirely clear. Currently, approximately 13 people per 100,000 are diagnosed with ulcerative colitis and 16 people per 100,000 are diagnosed with Crohn's disease.

IBD most commonly develops between ages 15 and 35. However, children as young as age 2 have been diagnosed with the disease. There's a second peak of diagnosis between ages 55 and 65.

IBD occurs equally in men and women. In Americans, it tends to occur more often in whites, particularly individuals of Jewish descent. However, more Blacks and Latinos are being diagnosed each year. In truth, there are no longer typical patients in terms of ethnicity. People living in all parts of the United States experience IBD. Globally, IBD tends to occur in industrialized nations rather than in developing countries and appears to be associated with better sanitation, for reasons that aren't understood.

WERE YOU MISDIAGNOSED?

Misdiagnosis is possible. Many symptoms of Crohn's disease and ulcerative colitis mimic other conditions. For instance, short-term inflammation in the gut may be caused by a bacterial, viral or parasitic infection. Taking medications like ibuprofen can cause pain, cramping and diarrhea associated with ulcers in the intestines that might be mistaken for ulcerative colitis or Crohn's disease. Sometimes blood tests will suggest IBD without other supporting information. (Receiving a correct diagnosis is discussed in greater detail in Chapters 2 and 3.)

In fact, there are a multitude of conditions that can act or look like IBD on diagnostic tests. In some individuals, IBD can be difficult to diagnose early on, and only after living with its symptoms for some time does it become apparent that chronic inflammation is occurring. In many cases, people have symptoms for almost two years before an accurate diagnosis is made.

IBD vs. IBS

It's easy to mix up IBD and irritable bowel syndrome (IBS). They occur in the same area of the body, and they often share similar symptoms, such as pain and diarrhea. They also typically develop at about the same age. But a thorough medical exam that includes diagnostic testing can make the distinction between IBD and IBS.

IBS is estimated to occur in 15% of the U.S. population, or about 50 million people. It's more common in women than in men. Although the cause of IBS is not completely understood, it appears to be related to problems with the nerves that control gut function. You may hear that a diagnosis of IBS is one of exclusion. This is because there are no specific tests for IBS; instead, a diagnosis is made using specific symptom criteria.

With IBS, there's no active inflammation of the GI tract, so there are no bouts of the bleeding or fever that are common with IBD. IBD is associated with chronic inflammation that sometimes flares up. Damage to the GI tract that occurs with IBD can be serious and requires treatment, whereas the symptoms of IBS can go away without treatment. It should be noted that some people with IBS struggle with almost constant digestive issues. While they can be quite disruptive, the symptoms aren't life-threatening.

It's also important to understand that having IBD doesn't make you immune to IBS. Studies suggest that as many as half of individuals diagnosed with Crohn's disease have IBS, and a third of people with ulcerative colitis have IBS.

Confirming your diagnosis

If you've received a diagnosis of IBD, you may want to consider seeing a doctor who's a specialist in this area. All gastroenterologists receive training in IBD, but some take a special interest in its diagnosis and management, just as others might specialize in diseases affecting the pancreas or liver. You may like and respect your own personal physician, but it never hurts to meet with someone who's up to date on IBD to confirm the diagnosis and review your current health and care plan, especially if you're not responding to treatment.

Remember, we're talking about a lifelong disease, and a correct diagnosis and the right treatment plan ultimately provide for the best outcomes. If you're worried about creating hard feelings, be sure to tell your doctor up front that you like and trust him or her and just want to include the viewpoint of an expert eye. Often, an IBD expert will co-manage your care with your personal physician.

IBD experts can be found in small private practices as well as large university medical centers. The Crohn's & Colitis Foundation (see page 183) is an excellent source of information and can help you find a physician who's a member of that organization and treats more people with IBD than perhaps other doctors in your community.

The future remains very bright for people with IBD. Researchers are actively working toward a cure. But in the meantime, there are ways to manage the disease and minimize its symptoms and side effects.

CLUES AS TO A CAUSE

There's no simple answer to the question of why you developed IBD. The reality is that we don't know why you got ulcerative colitis or Crohn's disease. Many popular theories have been proposed over the years that haven't panned out. They include eating refined sugar, drinking pasteurized milk, the use of refrigeration, the use of toothpaste and receiving the measles vaccine, just to name a few.

It's unlikely there's a simple answer. Research scientists believe that a combination of factors, including individual genetics, immune system responses and environmental triggers, may somehow come together to form the "perfect storm," resulting in IBD. Let's look at each of these factors more closely.

Genetics

So far, studying those genes associated with IBD has failed to reveal the role they play in development of the disease. IBD is different from disorders such as sickle cell disease or cystic fibrosis, in which a single gene is responsible for a specific mutation that leads to disease.

For a time, it seemed that the *NOD2* gene might be responsible for causing Crohn's disease. This was an extremely exciting discovery by two different investigators using two different techniques at the same time. The *NOD2* gene resembles a gene found in plants that helps them resist bacterial infection and resulting disease. In humans, the function of the *NOD2* gene is to help the body handle specific kinds of bacteria. A mutation or "defect" in this gene leads to impaired handling of these bacteria. It may be that an inability to handle bacteria, along with other factors that we've yet to fully understand, may uncover the final pathway of IBD. This is intriguing because one of the proposed theories regarding the cause of Crohn's disease is bacterial infection with a mycobacterium species (see page 21).

Scientists are actively studying several other genes that are associated with, but not a direct cause of, either Crohn's disease or ulcerative colitis: *IL23R, IRGM, ATG16L1 and TLR2, TLR3, TLR4, TLR5, TLR6 and TLR9*. These genes, when mutated, show up more often in patients with IBD. For instance, the *IRGM* and *ATG16L1* genes play a role in autophagy, which is the body's way of dealing with old and "broken" cells and a process that leads, eventually, to death. When the body is unable to correctly choose which cells should be alive and allowed to function and which need to be broken down and disposed of, this can lead to disease.

Most people who develop IBD don't necessarily have one or all of these defective genes. Only 8% to 17% of those diagnosed with Crohn's disease show evidence of having two abnormal *NOD2* genes; 27% to 32% have one abnormal *NOD2* gene. Furthermore, if you happen to carry one of these defective genes, you aren't destined to develop IBD. On the other hand, not having them doesn't make you immune to IBD. Therefore, it isn't particularly helpful to test for the presence of any of the mutated genes among patients.

An individual will often ask about the chance of getting Crohn's or ulcerative colitis if a family member has it. Although this may not be true for you, most people with IBD don't have a family member known to have the disease. People will also ask about the possibility of "passing it along" to children. In the strictest sense, IBD isn't a genetic disorder.

Factors other than genetics likely are involved in development of the disease.

Here are a few facts regarding heredity and IBD:
- Of individuals diagnosed, 30% have a family history of IBD.
- The chance of getting IBD if a family member has it is greatest if it's a first-degree relative (a parent or sibling), but your risk is still higher than the general population if the relative is second degree, like a cousin.
- The chance of passing IBD to your child is roughly 3% to 7%.
- If both parents have IBD, the chance of their child developing IBD increases to 45%. However, there's no specific recommendation that couples who both have IBD be counseled regarding having children, because IBD is not a genetic disease like sickle cell anemia or cystic fibrosis, in which counseling is commonly recommended.

Immune system

The human immune system, which keeps our bodies healthy by resisting foreign invaders, seems to play a starring role in IBD. The immune system is composed of cells that act in various ways, depending on what the body needs to do to defend itself. Sometimes, one of the protective things the body needs is inflammation. It could be that IBD occurs when the immune system overreacts to an infection or injury and keeps producing proteins that end up causing inflammation in the GI tract. Understanding how the immune system works may help you visualize what's happening in your body.

We'll consider both "innate" immunity and "humoral" immunity.

Some researchers believe that a defect in innate immunity causes IBD. Innate immunity is created by blood cells that respond within the first minute to an injury or infection, like a burn or insect bite. These cells are produced by the bone marrow.

The second line of defense is called humoral immunity, which involves cells that are called into action 24 hours after an insult, like an injury or infection. Examples of humoral immunity are the antibodies that your body makes after you receive a vaccination or after you've had an infection. Another type of humoral immunity involves the cells that form scar tissue to help heal wounds.

Some researchers believe that IBD is the result of an overreaction by humoral immunity. The cells involved in humoral immunity create certain substances such as proteins to fight infection or form scar tissue. Therapies we currently use to treat IBD mainly target the humoral immune system and get it to stop producing the specific proteins found in the blood and tissues of people with IBD.

Tumor necrosis factor (TNF), a humoral immune system protein, is an important target of therapy. TNF has become famous. It was first discovered in the blood of rats bred to develop large cancers to study the effects of different chemotherapies. That's why its name has the word tumor in it. It wasn't until much later that scientists figured out TNF isn't made by cancer cells but is produced by the body as part of a normal response to an insult.

Because TNF is powerful in causing inflammation, blocking the action of TNF is a successful therapy for many people with IBD as well as other inflammatory conditions. However, we don't want to completely shut off TNF action, because it assists in fighting off what the body identifies as foreign and helps decrease our risk of certain infections.

What's fascinating is that the terminal ileum — the last part of the small intestine just before it joins the colon — is where most of the immune activity for the gut happens, and that's the area most likely to be involved in Crohn's disease. In addition to the immune system, the body's lymph system assists in resisting and healing disease. There's lymphatic tissue throughout the GI tract, but most is located at the end of the small intestine.

Environment

There are two different environments, the one around us and the one within us. The environment around us is essentially the air we breathe and what we eat and drink. For example, we know that cigarette smokers are much more likely to develop Crohn's disease than nonsmokers and that cigarette smoking makes Crohn's disease worse. Our food or water also may contain substances that cause illness. For some people with food intolerances and allergies, exposure to a nutrient like lactose in milk produces inflammation of the GI tract, which results in cramping, bloating and diarrhea.

Food may contain organisms, such as bacteria, that upset the natural balance of bacteria in our gut. Taking antibiotics may also disrupt the natural bacterial balance of the gut. An infection with certain organisms can lead to chronic inflammation of the gut and make IBD worse. On the other hand, taking in more of the naturally occurring intestinal bacteria by drinking or eating probiotics may be helpful for some people with or without IBD. There's more information about this in Chapter 6.

The idea that a particular species of mycobacteria — *M. paratuberculosis* (MAP) — may be the cause of Crohn's disease is under active investigation. Researchers have been able to culture this bacterium from the tissue of some patients with Crohn's disease. It's found mainly in livestock and causes a condition in dairy cows that looks like Crohn's disease.

It's thought that MAP may be spread to humans via unpasteurized milk and perhaps through the air. In small studies, a course of antibiotics against MAP has successfully treated Crohn's symptoms in some people. However, no cause-and-effect relationship has been proven. To prove that MAP is the cause of Crohn's disease:

- MAP would need to be present in every person with Crohn's.
- Treatment of MAP would need to cure Crohn's completely.
- Infecting someone with MAP would need to cause Crohn's.

Obviously, we won't expose healthy people to MAP to see if they develop Crohn's disease. As tempting as it is to blame a single agent, and as much as we would like to believe it, there isn't enough evidence to say that MAP causes Crohn's disease. For now, we continue to believe that three important factors — your genetics, immune system and environment — interact to bring about Crohn's and other forms of IBD.

Lacking knowledge as to its exact cause, the only advice we can give about how to avoid IBD is to encourage individuals with a family history of Crohn's disease not to smoke, to eat a healthy diet and to limit use of anti-inflammatory medication, such as ibuprofen.

DEALING WITH YOUR FEELINGS

Quality-of-life studies indicate that most people with IBD feel about the same as those who don't have the disease. The exception is during bouts of inflammation when the disease is flaring. The unpredictability of disease symptoms and embarrassing problems like urgency, gas and loss of bowel control (fecal incontinence) definitely add to the burden of having IBD. Therefore, it's not surprising that studies suggest that more people with IBD experience signs and symptoms of depression than the general population. Unfortunately, depression in individuals with IBD often goes undiagnosed or untreated.

The five stages of grief, as described by Elisabeth Kübler-Ross, are applicable to IBD. Consider each of them on your own terms and in the context of where you are now. Doing this may help you appreciate what you're feeling, and that's the first step you need to take in self-management.

Denial

A typical response to the news that someone has IBD is, "This can't be Crohn's disease; it must be an infection or parasite." Individuals may visit several different doctors and hear the same thing. It's good to get a second opinion, especially from an institution that has special expertise in the diagnosis and management of IBD. It's when you've been to your fourth doctor and received the same response that it's time to accept the diagnosis and move on.

From individuals who've been diagnosed for some time, we commonly hear, "I don't think this is a flare. It's probably just something I ate or the flu." It's important to listen to your body and really think about whether your symptoms are consistent with a flare — and you just don't want to believe it — or whether you really have caught a flu bug going around the community or your office. The longer you deny active symptoms, the more likely you are to need more aggressive therapy to deal with their effects. It's better to face reality and be proactive than procrastinate and potentially create more problems for yourself.

EATING DISORDERS AND IBD

A special note here about eating disorders. There are times when people with Crohn's disease are diagnosed inappropriately with an eating disorder because their diets are so limited, whether it's their choice or disease induced.

We've seen individuals take it upon themselves to limit what they eat so severely that they could be classified as anorexic because of their aversion to food. Anorexia is a condition that can also go undiagnosed, as many health care providers assume that your Crohn's is keeping you underweight and malnourished. You may also get misdiagnosed as bulimic if it's noticed that you're in the bathroom all the time after a meal, whether to have a bowel movement or vomit.

That's why it is important to be honest with your health care providers about your symptoms and to share your diagnosis with the people who spend the most time with you.

Anger

"Why me? I don't deserve this!" Of course you don't. But being angry doesn't solve anything, nor is it a productive use of your time and energy. Many people have disabilities; some just hide them better than others. We tend to think that other people are perfect or have it all together, but it isn't true. The sooner you can stop being angry at yourself or the world, the sooner you can move on toward more positive behaviors.

Bargaining

"If I just eat better and give up smoking, this will all go away." This is spoken all the time. But it isn't true. Changing your diet can improve your symptoms and your overall health (see Chapter 10), but it may not stop the inflammatory process. Making beneficial lifestyle changes is absolutely a great response, but doing so won't make your IBD go away.

Depression

Depression is higher among people with IBD than in the general population, and it often goes undiagnosed or untreated. Being unable to work, socialize and eat what you want or being in constant pain can lead to situational depression or a prolonged depressive state. No one would necessarily blame you, but not doing anything about it is counterproductive. Sometimes treating depression is more important than treating the underlying disease.

Some antidepressants have potential side effects that may work to your advantage. Some stimulate the appetite and others have a constipating effect. Fortunately, there's no longer a stigma about being on an antidepressant, nor is it viewed as a weakness on your part if you need something to help improve your mood. Of more concern are some medications used to treat anxiety, which should be considered short-term therapy because they can be addictive.

Acceptance

The last stage of the grieving process is acceptance. This is when you can finally move on and take actions to help you get better. Sometimes you'll try things that don't work, but a positive attitude about your condition makes it easier to have open discussions with your health care providers about your concerns and issues. There are also good data to suggest that patients with positive attitudes respond better to therapies and overall have better outcomes.

TELLING OTHERS

Explaining IBD to others can be extremely difficult and traumatic. In addition, depending on whom you're trying to tell, the consequences can feel devastating. It's tricky when, on the outside, you look perfectly normal, but you're actually feeling quite terrible. It can be embarrassing to have to rush to the restroom throughout the day or explain why you can't accept a dinner invitation or go out to a social event because of how you need to eat.

Family members

It's important to let family members know you have IBD because of the genetic component. Having a family member with IBD places blood relatives at greater risk. It may be that your family members will be relieved when you tell them; they may have noticed long before you did that there was something wrong. Explain that while they may have an increased risk, this isn't an infectious disease, and they won't "catch it" from you.

Friends

It may be that your friends also noticed signs that you didn't seem well, and if they're really friends, they'll be supportive about your disclosure. Not telling them can lead to hard feelings and misunderstandings if you continually decline invitations or leave early from events. They may think that you don't want to spend time with them! You'll be surprised by how many people, upon learning that you have ulcerative colitis or Crohn's disease, will say, "Boy, I know so-and-so with it, too," or even more shocking, "I have it, too, and never told anyone."

Potential partners

Dating can be such a stressful activity, and the timing of when to tell someone you're dating that you have ulcerative colitis or Crohn's can be tough. Part of how a potential partner may take the news is informed by how you met: Were you set up by friends who knew of your condition, or was your meeting at random or from an online source? Sometimes the situation arises before you want it to, like having to run for a bathroom when you aren't prepared. That may actually be the perfect time to share the information, as you can use the event as the springboard to a conversation regarding your diagnosis.

The timing for a such a conversation shouldn't necessarily be on the first date, but neither do you want to wait so long only to find out you've invested time in someone who turns out to be unaccepting of your condition. A lot of it depends on your personality, how open you are with others and how accepting you are of others' shortcomings.

Remember that no one is perfect, no matter how they appear. We all face challenges, and yours is IBD. Examples we've heard suggest having a discussion around the third or fourth date that starts off something like, "Do you wonder why I stay away from the salad bar when we go out to eat? Well …" or, "It may seem like I spend a lot more time in the bathroom than some of your other friends. It isn't because I'm vain, but …"

Coworkers, boss, employer

The workplace is another tough situation. On the one hand, you don't want people to feel sorry for you or discriminate against you because of your condition. On the other hand, you want people to understand and be somewhat more forgiving if you're having a bad day, week or even month.

Your health care provider may be able to help in this instance, with a letter to your employer or boss that could pave the way for certain accommodations, like having your desk near a bathroom or limiting how much weight you're required to lift. In return, however, you have to be willing to meet people halfway and perform your duties to the best of your abilities, so that no one begrudges your "special favors." Perhaps you don't want special favors, but having someone at work who understands your situation will be an advantage on days when you can't perform at your best.

Understanding ulcerative colitis

Ulcerative colitis is chronic inflammation of the innermost lining of the colon. Chronic means long term, lasting more than six weeks. This inflammation often leads to diarrhea, bleeding, cramping and urgency. No one understands exactly why ulcerative colitis occurs. There are many theories. As discussed in Chapter 1, it's doubtful one thing alone causes ulcerative colitis. Instead, it's likely to be a combination of genes, environment and something else that triggers the body to initiate the inflammation process and not shut it off as it's supposed to.

Once the inflammation process has been turned on, it can be difficult to get it turned off, so we aim to control it. Stopping it would amount to curing it. Many scientists are searching for this cure.

In virtually 100% of people with ulcerative colitis, inflammation starts in the rectum, and over time, it may progress up through the colon. Some people experience inflammation only in the rectum; this form of ulcerative colitis is called ulcerative proctitis to refer to the fact that only the rectum is inflamed. It would be clearer if we called this problem ulcerative "rectitis," but in medicine, we use the Latin term for rectum, which is procto.

When the left side of the colon is involved in the inflammation, we call it left-sided ulcerative colitis, and when the entire colon is involved, we call it pancolitis. When first diagnosed, you may have proctitis or left-sided colitis, but over time, the inflammation may progress to involve the entire colon. This progression usually happens within the first two years after diagnosis.

Ask the doctor who diagnosed your condition if biopsies were taken from throughout the entire colon. Sometimes, when things look typical, doctors tend not to biopsy those areas. However, under the microscope, there may be evidence of subtle inflammation that over time may reveal itself. You may then feel like your colitis spread when, actually, it was there all along but not readily visible.

SYMPTOMS OF ULCERATIVE COLITIS

Certain predictable problems occur when the lining of the colon is inflamed.

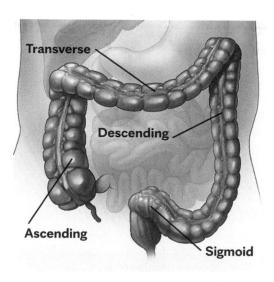

The large intestine (colon) almost completely frames the small intestine. The colon is shorter than the small intestine, but its diameter is greater. It's divided into sections, as shown.

Because the parts of the colon that are inflamed no longer absorb water, the most common problem is diarrhea. Water that's no longer being absorbed comes out with the stool.

If the inflammation continues or becomes worse, it causes the innermost lining of the colon to break down. This damage is called ulceration and is similar to what your skin looks like when you fall down and scrape yourself. You end up with a break in the skin and some bleeding, depending on how hard you fell. These ulcerations bleed, so blood appears in your stool.

Inflammation also breaks the normal communication between colon and brain that indicates when you need to have a bowel movement. The rectum contains stretch receptors that detect how full it is. Healthy receptors don't detect a stretch until a regular-size stool is present and is ready to be excreted by way of a bowel movement.

Inflammation temporarily damages these stretch signals. It makes them hypersensitive. The result is that whether there's stool or only air in the rectum, the signal is sent that you need to pass stool and you need to do it right now! You're not able to tell the difference. When you go to the bathroom and pass just gas or a little mucus or blood, you might have what some doctors call dry heaves of the rectum.

The medical term for this is tenesmus. Not being able to sense the difference between gas, mucus, blood or stool in the rectum can lead to false alarms that send you rushing to the bathroom.

Many people with ulcerative colitis say they have to go the bathroom more often in the morning and that the need decreases throughout the day. We call this the "morning rush hour," and it's natural because we possess reflexes that make the bowels most active within the first few hours after getting up. Understanding this phenomenon — that the majority of your bowel movements are likely to happen in the first one to two hours after getting out of bed in the morning — may make it easier to plan your day.

Along with diarrhea, urgency and bleeding, you may experience cramps, which tend to worsen around the time you have to move your bowels because the colon muscles are contracting. Cramps generally get better within a few minutes following bowel evacuation. Cramps can be severe but normally aren't long lasting.

Because pain fibers are located on the outside of the bowel and ulcerative colitis affects the inner lining of the bowel, nerves that sense pain generally don't become irritated. However, you may experience pain in the anal area from frequent bowel movements and the breakdown of normal perianal skin. This is due to stool frequency and diarrhea and not inflammation.

Other symptoms can include nighttime bowel movements, fever, loss of appetite and weight loss. In Chapter 7 you'll learn about other parts of the body that can exhibit inflammation associated with ulcerative colitis.

If your ulcerative colitis is confined to the rectum (proctitis), constipation can be more of an issue than diarrhea. This is because when the rectum is inflamed, the rest of the colon tends to slow passage of waste to assist the rectum by letting it rest. Patients with proctitis generally experience constipation, passing blood alone and passing bright-red blood along with relatively solid stools.

When ulcerative colitis is particularly severe — during periods of intense inflammation — you may experience fever, constant cramping and abdominal discomfort, along with a sense of bloating or abdominal swelling. Stools may be frequent — up to one every hour — and contain blood. Nausea and vomiting may also occur if the colon is severely inflamed.

In all but rare circumstances, this situation requires hospitalization for close monitoring by health care professionals. Dehydration is dangerous and can occur quickly, and you'll need medications and intravenous fluids to keep you safe.

DIAGNOSING ULCERATIVE COLITIS

Health care providers diagnose ulcerative colitis using a combination of a detailed medical history, physical examination and testing. A thorough medical history consists of your answers to many questions to rule out other types of colitis. Tests are usually stool studies, blood work and an endoscopic procedure.

Medical history

For your medical history, the more detailed information you can provide, the better.

- When did you first notice the symptoms? (In other words, how long has this been going on?)
- Are your symptoms getting worse or just not going away?
- Have you started or stopped any new medications recently, including supplements, vitamins and other over-the-counter (nonprescription) therapies?
- Have you traveled outside your normal environment?
- Does anyone with whom you've been in recent contact have similar symptoms?
- Have you recently quit smoking?
- Do you have family members who have ulcerative colitis or Crohn's disease?
- Have you had any rashes, joint aches or eye problems along with your bowel symptoms?

Tests

Blood tests usually include a complete blood count (CBC) to check for anemia and evidence of infection; a chemistry panel (CMP) to check electrolytes, kidney and liver function, and protein levels; and a sedimentation rate or C-reactive protein (CRP) test, two common tests that indicate active inflammation.

There are blood tests that can look for special proteins associated with the presence of either Crohn's disease or ulcerative colitis. These tests, however, should never be performed in the absence of other testing, because the information they provide isn't sufficient to diagnose either disease. They can be helpful in two situations. The first is when you've been diagnosed with IBD and physicians are trying to determine if you have Crohn's disease or ulcerative colitis. The other is in determining inflammation aggressiveness in young individuals.

Stool tests look for white blood cells or specific proteins that indicate inflammation, as well as the presence of certain bacteria, parasites or toxins that could explain your symptoms. Yeast, in particular *Candida*, is typical in stool and doesn't indicate a disease. A stool test called calprotectin is being used more frequently in patients with known IBD to monitor inflammation over time once treatment begins.

Colonoscopy

A diagnosis of ulcerative colitis requires evidence of inflammation in the colon or rectum. This evidence is collected by viewing the inside of the colon and rectum and taking samples (biopsies) of the colon lining.

During a colonoscopy, a doctor examines the entire colon. You must prepare for this exam the day before by consuming a clear liquid diet and drinking a cleansing solution. Some procedures, such as a flexible sigmoidoscopy, can be done in the office without any prep or sedatives. This shorter exam involves only the lower third to bottom half of the colon. It doesn't require an oral prep and usually involves one or two enemas. Sometimes no prep is needed, in the case of severe diarrhea when there's no solid stool to clean out.

If you've never had a colonoscopy, know that the prep is actually the roughest part of the procedure. Bowel cleansing is important for a complete and thorough

COLON CLEANSING PREPARATIONS

Name	Form	Comment
GoLYTELY	1 gallon fluid	Effective agents in general use
NuLYTELY	½ gallon fluid	
MoviPrep	½ gallon fluid	
Colyte	1 gallon fluid	
HalfLytely	½ gallon fluid	
TriLyte	1 gallon fluid	
SUPREP	½ gallon fluid	
PLENVU	½ gallon fluid	
OsmoPrep	32 tablets	Phosphorous-based and can lead to kidney problems; not recommended
SUTAB	24 tablets	Sodium sulfate, magnesium sulfate and potassium chloride-based
Magnesium citrate + modified diet	Multiple bottles over 12 to 16 hours	Carefully following directions is essential for adequate prep
Prepopik	10 oz fluid plus eight 8-oz glasses of water	
MiraLAX and Gatorade	A full bottle of MiraLAX and non-red Gatorade	Well tolerated and over the counter, but not the most effective prep

look at the lining of the colon. Cleansing is generally split into two parts: You take some of the preparation the night before your procedure and the rest the morning of the procedure, several hours before you arrive. Splitting the dose of laxative has been shown to produce better-prepped colons, allowing for better views.

The table on the opposite page shows the different preparation formulations available. All generally taste bad because they contain a lot of salt that's not absorbed, causing water to be excreted from the colon wall to create diarrhea and flush out (cleanse) the colon of all stool.

These salts aren't the same as table salt, so there's no need to worry about your blood pressure going up when you use them. Some doctors have invented their own cocktail of agents they feel is more palatable, including some that combine Gatorade and powdered laxatives. Ask your physician what formulation he or she prefers and why. That might help you understand the formulation prescribed for you.

Sedative medications will keep you comfortable during the procedure. Sedatives are safer than general anesthesia. Because you aren't totally out, you don't need a breathing tube and recovery is easier. Conscious sedation typically involves the medication midazolam, which is like a fast-acting diazepam (Valium), along with the drug fentanyl. Some people instead choose monitored anesthesia administered by specially trained providers, which involves a

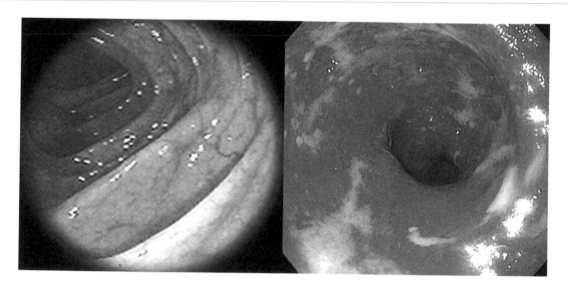

The image at left shows typical folding and tissue coloration in the transverse colon. The image at right reveals ulcerative colitis with ulcerations. The inflammation develops only in the thin lining of the inner surface.

deeper level of sedation using the medication propofol. If you're concerned, talk to your doctor before the procedure to find out the level of sedation and medications used. The goal is to have a safe and comfortable procedure.

A colonoscopy takes about 20 minutes, but it may be longer depending on the length of your colon, how twisted it is inside your abdominal cavity and how many biopsies are being taken. Among women, the colon tends to be curvier than in men because it has to divert around the uterus. Women may have a little more discomfort than men during a colonoscopy. Most people tolerate it well.

For this procedure, a thin, flexible tube called a colonoscope is inserted into the colon by way of the rectum. The colonoscope contains a light and video camera, along with tiny attached instruments. The doctor conducting the exam carefully passes the scope through the colon until it reaches the cecum and the end of the small intestine.

Along the way, small pinches of tissue (biopsies) are gathered from the inner lining of the colon. The biopsies are later examined under a microscope by a pathologist for evidence of inflammation, which is essential for a correct diagnosis. Examination of the tissue under a microscope also helps eliminate other conditions that can sometimes look like ulcerative colitis.

It's important for you to have at least one colonoscopy in which your entire colon is examined and biopsied to find all areas of inflammation.

When inflammation of the entire colon is severe, the end of the small intestine (terminal ileum) also may show signs of inflammation. This is because the valve that separates the colon from the terminal ileum may weaken, and inflammation "backwashes" into the ileum. We call this backwash ileitis, which suggests an active, highly inflamed case of ulcerative colitis.

Making a diagnosis in older adults

As you learned in Chapter 1, IBD can affect individuals of all ages and backgrounds. Among older individuals, however, diagnosing and managing the condition can be more complex. That's because many older adults often aren't as healthy as they once were.

Although IBD is most often diagnosed in young people, it isn't as rare in older adults as previously thought. There's a second, smaller peak of IBD diagnoses between ages 55 and 65. Up to 20% of people with ulcerative colitis or Crohn's disease are older when they begin experiencing symptoms. This is a special population with its own set of challenges, beginning with the mistaken idea that IBD doesn't happen to older people.

There are other obstacles to reaching a correct diagnosis of IBD. In someone who has diabetes or other conditions, symptoms caused by those conditions can get mixed up with possible symptoms of IBD. In addition, people may present with

Pat is 75 years old, is very overweight, and has high cholesterol and high blood pressure. She was recently diagnosed with type 2 diabetes and is facing hip replacement surgery. Over the past year, she's had episodes of diarrhea and fecal incontinence, requiring her to wear adult diapers if she's away from home for any length of time. She's always been a hearty eater, continues to enjoy her favorite foods and hasn't been able to single out which ones might be triggering her distressing condition. Pat is a widow, lives alone and has some money concerns, but her sons and their families live nearby.

different symptoms depending on their age. So, we can't always be clear about what's going on because we don't yet have universal diagnostic criteria that apply equally well to people of all ages.

When doctors see an older adult with new symptoms suggestive of IBD, such as bloody diarrhea or abdominal pain, we compile a thorough medical history and then consider other conditions and factors, including medication use, that can produce similar symptoms.

Conditions a doctor may want to rule out include:
- A bacterial, viral or parasitic infection.
- Ischemic colitis, caused by lack of blood flow to the colon that damages its lining.
- Microscopic colitis, normal-appearing tissue that's actually inflamed when viewed under a microscope.
- Radiation colitis, damage to the colon from administration of radiation to treat cancer, including prostate cancer and cervical cancer.
- Diverticular disease, formation of small pouches in the colon wall.
- Cancer.

- Medication use, including use of nonsteroidal anti-inflammatory drugs (NSAIDs).

Atypical symptoms are more common in older adults. Natural aging also must be considered. For example, involuntary release of stool (fecal incontinence) is more of an issue with advancing age due to weakness of the anal sphincter muscles. This is especially true in women who had vaginal deliveries during childbirth.

Doctors often need help tracking symptoms, although this can be a challenge in some older individuals. The presence of other conditions, such as coronary artery disease, high blood pressure, peripheral vascular disease or diabetes, may mean that older adults with IBD are much sicker than younger individuals usually are. That's why older adults are more often hospitalized when they receive a diagnosis, to make sure they're getting all the care they need.

Pat, whose story is above, did indeed have ulcerative colitis. But her disease didn't respond as well as hoped to the medication she was first prescribed, and she was forced to take steroids. (See Chapter 6 for information about medications to treat ulcerative colitis.) The steroids made her diabetes worse, and she required additional insulin until her colitis was under control. She then returned to her initial medication, which she's tolerated well. Pat is happy that once again she's able to sit through a bridge game without having to make several trips to the bathroom.

MANAGING ULCERATIVE COLITIS

You may have experienced symptoms for months, perhaps years, before you eventually received a diagnosis. Once diagnosed, however, treatment can begin. One rule of thumb is that, in many cases, the length of time you've been sick is about how long it may take you to get better. There are very few quick fixes.

Your treatment needs to be individualized to your specific needs. Factors to consider may include:
- Where in the colon the inflammation is located.
- The severity and extent of the inflammation.
- Whether you have a history of allergies.
- Your insurance coverage (every insurance company has preferred medications that may differ from what your physician wants to prescribe).
- Your other medical conditions.
- Your personal preferences.

Therapy for ulcerative colitis is definitely not one-size-fits-all. Two people with the same set of symptoms and severity may be treated in completely different ways,

depending on other individual factors. However, management goals are the same for everyone, regardless of individual circumstances. The three main goals of treatment are:
- Getting your symptoms under control as quickly and as safely as possible.
- Keeping your symptoms under control.
- Confirming that the inflammation in your colon has resolved or at least improved.

While there is no cure for ulcerative colitis, there are medications that can decrease your symptoms. Chapter 6 details the medications used to treat ulcerative colitis. Know that with proper treatment, it's possible to heal the colon lining so that it looks typical and isn't inflamed, even at the level visible only under a microscope.

In determining the best treatment, doctors take into consideration the location of the inflammation as well as the severity of the disease. Someone with only a few inches of disease in the colon can be worse off than someone with mild symptoms involving the entire colon.

When several courses of steroids are required to control symptoms, this is often the tipping point that signals the need for more aggressive therapy. Make sure you've discussed with your health care provider an exit strategy to get you off the steroids once you've started them.

In addition to medication, in some cases surgery may be required to manage symptoms and control the disease. Surgery is discussed in Chapter 9.

Michael is 31 years old and had been having loose stools for the past six months. He didn't think much about his bowel habits, because having to go frequently didn't keep him from his work or other daily activities. But then he started to notice blood in his stool. At first, he thought it was hemorrhoids because he didn't have any abdominal pain. Once he started to experience some abdominal cramping, he decided to seek medical advice. His doctor sent him for a colonoscopy, after which he was told he had ulcerative colitis. Michael was started on medications and got better fairly quickly. After a few weeks, he stopped taking the medications. After all, no one had told him that he had to continue taking them if his symptoms were better. Unfortunately, within a few months' time, his symptoms returned, and he found himself back where he started.

Flares

Many people will say, "I've been feeling well for such a long time that I don't need my medicine anymore." We wish that were true. For most people, if they stop taking their medication, their symptoms will eventually return. We call these flares.

It's true that some people can go into remission and stay off their medicines, for even up to a few years. Unfortunately, this is a small minority of people; for most, their ulcerative colitis will flare up again. A recent internet survey of people with ulcerative colitis revealed that, on average, they have six to eight flares per year. However, only a fraction are reported to their doctors. Most people treat the flares on their own and don't necessarily recognize a pattern of repeated flares.

Not all flares stem from stopping or reducing ulcerative colitis medications.

There are other culprits. Use of certain antibiotics can cause a flare. If you're prescribed antibiotics, discuss with the doctor why they're necessary. Some antibiotics are safer than others for people with inflammatory bowel disease; if you must take them, make sure you receive those least likely to be harmful.

Flares can occur while traveling, when your normal routine is disrupted. Other causes include an acute illness, such as the flu or a sinus infection. Many people report a seasonal variation in their symptoms, particularly spring and fall (April and October, respectively, in the United States). We aren't entirely sure why this occurs, but it's a well-documented phenomenon.

Stopping smoking can make ulcerative colitis worse and may trigger a flare — a connection that baffles the medical community. People with ulcerative colitis are more likely to be ex-smokers or nonsmokers. And then there's stress, an important factor covered further in Chapter 11.

It's important to view your ulcerative colitis as a chronic condition, similar to diabetes or high blood pressure. There is no cure, but you can control it with medicines and healthy lifestyle choices. The more you know, the better you'll become at managing the condition to keep it from controlling your life.

3

Understanding Crohn's disease

Melissa is 28 years old and has had "stomach problems" since childhood. Her first surprise was to learn that she was anemic, although everyone assumed it was due to her menstrual periods. But when she started experiencing severe abdominal pain, she decided to see a doctor. A computerized tomography (CT) scan showed thickening of her small intestine, and a colonoscopy showed inflammation in her right colon and terminal ileum. Melissa was diagnosed with ileocolonic Crohn's disease. This was devastating news, as the only exposure she had to Crohn's disease was a close friend's mother, who had struggled with the disease for many years. Upset and scared, Melissa had a lot to learn about her disease and how it fit into her hopeful outlook for a full, long life.

Crohn's disease differs from ulcerative colitis in two important ways. Inflammation associated with Crohn's disease can occur throughout the digestive tract — both the small and large intestines. The inflammation involves all the layers of the intestinal wall. Ulcerative colitis is limited to the large intestine (colon) and involves only the inner layer of tissue.

In about one-third of people with Crohn's disease, inflammation is limited to the small intestine. Another third has inflammation in both the small intestine and colon. Among the last third, inflammation is confined to the colon. Regardless of where the inflammation is located, it can penetrate all layers of the intestinal wall as it progresses.

TYPES OF CROHN'S DISEASE

There are three types of Crohn's disease — inflammatory, fistulizing, and fibrostenosing. Almost everyone with Crohn's disease begins with inflammatory Crohn's that's limited to some portion of the gastrointestinal tract. Among many individuals, the disease remains in this inflammatory state.

Over time, about 30% of individuals experience inflammation that burrows through all layers of the intestinal wall and causes an abnormal connection (fistula) to another part of the body. This is known as fistulizing Crohn's.

Fistulas can develop between your intestine and your skin or between your intestine and another organ. Fistulas near

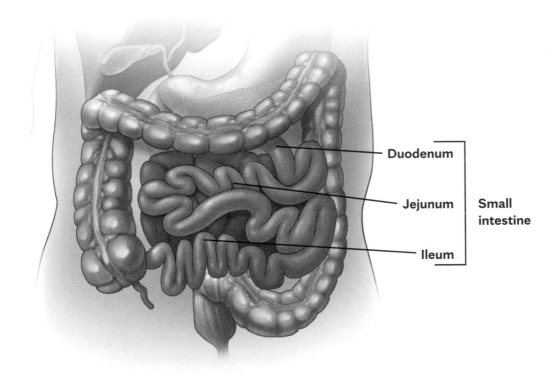

Crohn's disease can develop in the small or large intestine and may occur in both.

or around the anal area (perianal) are the most common kind. When fistulas develop in the abdomen, food may bypass areas of the bowel that are necessary for absorption, resulting in weight loss and diarrhea. Fistulas may form between loops of bowel, in the bladder or vagina, or through the skin, causing continuous drainage of bowel contents to your skin.

The third type of Crohn's occurs when inflammation continues to "smolder" over time. Scar tissue builds up and creates a thickening that causes narrowing (stenosis) of parts of the digestive tract. This fibrostenosing happens in about 30% of people with Crohn's disease at some point in their lives.

Medical providers also label the types of Crohn's disease by location and character. For example, someone with disease that's limited to inflammation in the large intestine would have Crohn's colitis. Someone with inflammation in the small intestine and no evidence of narrowing or fistula would be said to have inflammatory Crohn's ileitis. Someone with a fistula between the small intestine and colon with inflammation in both locations would have fistulizing ileocolitis.

SYMPTOMS OF CROHN'S DISEASE

Symptoms associated with Crohn's disease vary widely, depending on the location of the inflammation, how severe it is, and even your own perception of the symptoms. Signs and symptoms can range from mild to severe. They usually develop gradually, but on occasion will come on suddenly, without warning.

Because the most common location for Crohn's is at the end of the small intestine, the most common symptoms are generally abdominal pain, diarrhea that can occur during the day and at night, fatigue, nausea and sometimes vomiting, along with weight loss. Most people with small intestinal Crohn's disease don't experience any visible bleeding.

As the disease persists, weight loss, fever and joint pain may develop. Pediatricians might diagnose a child with Crohn's as a failure to grow. This is often the first sign of Crohn's disease in children.

Seventeen-year-old Sharon was experiencing pain after meals, which she described as crampy or sharp and usually on the right lower side of her abdomen. One night it got so bad that her parents brought her to the emergency department at their local hospital. Because of the location of the pain, doctors suspected she had appendicitis and ordered a CT scan of her abdomen. Sharon's appendix looked normal, but the last few inches of the small intestine (terminal ileum) were swollen and inflamed, suggesting she might have Crohn's disease.

Crohn's disease in the upper small intestines, or jejunum, usually results in pain in the middle of the abdomen, with associated bloating, gas and watery diarrhea. Involvement of the stomach can cause ulcers.

For Crohn's disease that occurs in the esophagus, which is relatively uncommon, symptoms may include difficult swallowing or pain with swallowing. The wide variety of symptoms can make the disease difficult to diagnose.

DIAGNOSING CROHN'S DISEASE

Because symptoms of Crohn's disease aren't specific and can manifest from many different conditions, medical evaluation is necessary to make the correct diagnosis.

The process starts with a complete medical history and physical exam. The more detailed and complete your history and list of symptoms that you can share with your health care provider, the better. You may be asked:

- When did you first notice the symptoms? (In other words, how long has this been going on?)
- Are your symptoms getting worse, or just not going away?
- Have you started or stopped any new medications recently, including supplements, vitamins and other nonprescription therapies?
- Have you traveled outside your normal environment?
- Does anyone with whom you've been in recent contact have similar symptoms?
- What surgeries have you had?
- Are you a smoker?
- Has anyone in your family been diagnosed with ulcerative colitis or Crohn's disease?
- Have you had any rashes, joint aches or eye problems along with your bowel symptoms?

Tad, a 20-year-old college student, was always small for his age. Being more of a computer nerd than an athlete, this didn't bother him. What did bother him, however, were big meals. After eating, he would experience bloating with visible swelling of his abdomen; loose, runny stools; and nausea. When he started college and watched his friends eat, he realized that he wasn't overeating after all. Even normal portions of food affected him, and once he realized this, he made a visit to the student health clinic at his college. It turned out that Tad had Crohn's disease of the small intestine, and his being small was really growth failure caused by damage to his small intestine. His inability to eat large meals came from scarring and narrowing of the intestine that caused blockages when he ate.

Physical exam

Following your medical history, you'll likely have a complete physical, examining your entire body, even those parts seemingly not involved with your symptoms. Your provider is looking for clues to what's causing your symptoms.

A rectal exam is typically part of a physical because many people with Crohn's disease have skin tags around the anus, which they may mistakenly self-diagnose as hemorrhoids. These skin tags can cause anal discomfort. Narrowing or cracks in the anal canal (fissures) can also be clues to Crohn's disease. On occasion, the first manifestation of Crohn's disease may be a perianal abscess (collection of pus) or a boil.

Sometimes a rectal exam is performed while you're sedated during a colonoscopy, so that the examination can be more thorough.

Tests

Your doctor will decide what tests to request based on the location of your symptoms. Most everyone starts with basic blood tests that include a complete blood count (CBC); iron studies to rule out an iron deficiency; a chemistry panel to assess electrolytes, kidney and liver function, and protein levels; evaluation of thyroid hormone levels; and a sedimentation rate or C-reactive protein test, two common tests that indicate active inflammation.

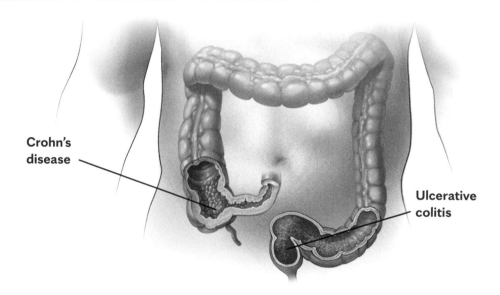

Crohn's disease

Ulcerative colitis

With Crohn's disease, the inflammation extends deep into the intestinal walls. Ulcerative colitis is confined to the innermost layer of tissue.

Some tests look for special proteins (markers) associated with the presence of either Crohn's disease or ulcerative colitis. These blood tests, however, should never be done in the absence of other testing because they don't provide enough information to diagnose either Crohn's disease or ulcerative colitis.

However, as we discuss in Chapter 2, they can be helpful in trying to determine which condition — Crohn's disease or ulcerative colitis — a person has. Another situation in which the tests are helpful is in determining the aggressiveness of the inflammation in young individuals.

These markers are proteins directed to act against bacteria, and antibodies directed to act against certain carbohydrates found in the body. These carbohydrates aren't the kind found in food but rather sugars that the body uses for energy. It's unclear why the body would react to specific carbohydrates, and their overall significance in the inflammatory disease process is unknown. Use of these markers is still in the research phase, so they aren't applicable to standard care.

Doctors also request stool studies to look for blood, bacteria, parasites and the toxin produced by the bacterium C. difficile. (See page 73 for more on C. difficile.) Stool may also be checked for fat content, which can suggest whether fat is being properly absorbed by the small intestine, or white blood cells, signaling inflammation.

Finally, your stool sample will be used to measure protein content. Certain pro-teins appear in the stool when inflammation is active. Calprotectin and lactoferrin are proteins that are such sensitive markers of inflammation that if they're absent in stool, we can be certain that no inflammation is occurring.

Imaging

Of course, it's essential to examine the digestive tract. Several tools are available to help doctors see what is happening inside.

Barium studies

Barium is a mixture that you swallow. It contains a substance that coats the digestive tract to help make key structures visible. With traditional barium studies, X-rays are taken of the digestive tract that may highlight obstructions or abnormalities. Barium studies are old-fashioned and outdated but still can serve a purpose in rare situations, such as outlining a long narrowing of the intestine (stricture).

Computerized tomography (CT)

This test looks at the entire bowel as well as at tissues outside the bowel. CT enterography (CTE) is a special CT scan that provides better images of the small bowel. This test has replaced barium X-rays in the overwhelming majority of medical centers. For most CT scans, including CTE, you still need to drink a contrast dye, although it's a thinner

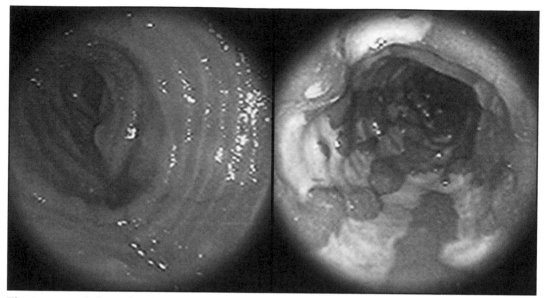

The image at left is a healthy small intestine with even coloration and well-spaced circular folds. The image at right shows the small intestine with a pattern of inflammation characteristic of Crohn's disease. The mucous membrane lining the interior of the small intestine forms bumpy nodules.

formula than used in the past. CTE allows doctors to really focus on details of the small intestinal wall.

Magnetic resonance imaging (MRI)

An MRI scanner uses a magnetic field and radio waves to create detailed images of organs and tissues. MRI is particularly useful for evaluating a fistula around the anal area (pelvic MRI) or the small intestine (MR enterography).

Colonoscopy

This test allows your doctor to view your entire colon and the end of your small intestine (terminal ileum) using a thin, flexible, lighted tube equipped with a camera located at the end. During the procedure, your doctor can also take small samples of tissue (biopsy) for laboratory analysis, which may help make a diagnosis.

Capsule endoscopy

For this test, you swallow a capsule about the size of a large vitamin pill that contains a camera. The camera takes pictures of your small intestine and transmits them to a recorder you wear on your belt. The images are downloaded to a computer and displayed on a monitor, and doctors study them like a movie. The camera can be quite sensitive, and even small ulcers and breaks in the small intestine lining can be seen. The camera exits your body painlessly in your stool. You may still need an endoscopy procedure with biopsies to confirm the diagnosis of Crohn's disease.

Balloon-assisted enteroscopy

This technique is useful when capsule endoscopy shows abnormalities but the diagnosis is still in question. A scope is used in conjunction with a device called an overtube, which enables a doctor to look farther into the small intestine, where standard endoscopes don't reach.

How does your doctor decide what test to use? It depends on the stage of your diagnosis and what your doctor is looking for. You might think of it this way. A regular CT scan lets doctors look at the whole body as if flying over the Grand Canyon in a commercial jet. They get an idea of how big it is but not a lot of detail. A CT scan with a contrast dye is like seeing the Grand Canyon from a helicopter — in much more detail and closer up. Colonoscopy or capsule endoscopy would be like being on the Colorado River in a raft where you're actually inside the Canyon.

So, what are doctors hoping to find on imaging tests? They're looking for several problems:
- There is evidence of inflammation or swelling of the wall of the intestine.
- Craters in the intestine wall, which can signal the presence of ulcers.

- Tracks of contrast dye outside the bowel, which may indicate an abnormal connection between two body parts (fistula).
- A narrowing of the intestine, which suggests an obstruction (stenosis).
- There is an area above a narrowing that's dilated from chronic stretching of the bowel due to stool having to sit before it can move through the narrow area.

MANAGING CROHN'S DISEASE

The nature of Crohn's disease is that it waxes and wanes. This means that there are periods of active disease (the waxing or buildup) interspersed with periods of disease remission (the waning).

The goal is to maximize the amount of time you spend in remission and minimize the number and duration of flares. This is generally achieved with medication and lifestyle changes. Medications to treat Crohn's disease are discussed in detail in Chapter 6.

Keep in mind that if you've been sick for some time before receiving your diagnosis and starting treatment, it may take a fair amount of time for you to reach a period of remission. There are few quick fixes with IBD.

How often you have flares and how long they last depend on several factors. While flares can seem to come on randomly, there are several known triggers. Stopping your medication will lead to flares. If the medication you're taking is keeping your disease in remission, then you need to stay on it.

It's important to understand that Crohn's disease is a chronic illness. Just like diabetes, Crohn's can't be cured, but it can be treated. For people who take insulin to treat their diabetes, a blood glucose reading in the normal range doesn't mean they should stop taking their insulin. It means that the treatment is working, and they should continue with their existing drug regimen.

Certain antibiotics can also cause a flare, including the group of antibiotics in the penicillin family. A disruption in your normal routine, such as traveling, may cause a flare. So can contracting an illness such as the flu or a sinus infection. Smoking makes Crohn's disease worse, so it's important to quit (or never start) smoking. The role of stress in the development of flares is controversial and discussed in Chapter 11.

Contrary to what you may have heard or read, Crohn's disease doesn't spread. In reality, within the first year of diagnosis, Crohn's disease is present in whatever part of the body it's going to affect. If, after a year, other parts of the GI tract suddenly develop symptoms, you may be certain that the disease already existed in those locations. They may not have been fully evaluated on diagnosis because there weren't any obvious signs of the disease.

When surgery has been performed on an individual with Crohn's disease, the disease typically recurs exactly where it was before. So, in that sense, it hasn't spread (see Chapter 9). We've yet to understand how Crohn's recurs after a piece of affected bowel is removed.

You know your body better than anyone else does. If you're experiencing symptoms that involve the GI tract but feel different from your usual flare, speak up. Having Crohn's disease doesn't make you immune to developing other illnesses, such as food poisoning, the stomach flu or a side effect from a medication.

For example, let's say you have Crohn's disease in your colon and a normal flare for you involves diarrhea and bleeding. But one day you develop nausea and vomiting. Nausea and vomiting are common symptoms of IBD, but you shouldn't automatically assume they're related to your Crohn's. This is a common mistake. We've even delayed a diagnosis of pregnancy in a young woman with persistent nausea because we were so focused on her Crohn's disease!

Other types of IBD

Crohn's disease and ulcerative colitis are the most common forms of IBD, but they aren't the only ones. Inflammation that presents itself in other ways also can affect the large and small intestines.

INDETERMINATE COLITIS

About 10% of people with IBD in the colon have what we call indeterminate colitis. This means that they have features of both Crohn's disease and ulcerative colitis. But it doesn't mean that they have both diseases.

If you've been diagnosed with indeterminate colitis, you have inflammation of the colon that's difficult to distinguish between the two diagnoses. Sometimes even experts have a hard time determin-

ing what's Crohn's disease and what's ulcerative colitis.

Remember, the term *colitis* simply means inflammation of the colon. Most people use the term *colitis* to refer to ulcerative colitis, but Crohn's disease of the colon is still colitis — it's Crohn's colitis. Management is typically the same regardless of which name you give it.

Sometimes, over the span of years, the colitis declares itself as either ulcerative colitis or Crohn's disease because its nature or the character of the symptoms changes somehow. However, studies show that people with indeterminate colitis continue to have features of both diseases that never really change, even after seven to 10 years of having the disease.

Jennifer, who is 24, began to notice a change in her bowel habits a few years ago. She saw blood in her stools and had some weight loss, along with cramping and diarrhea. A colonoscopy revealed inflammation throughout her entire colon, but her rectum looked pretty typical. Some of the ulcers noted were very deep, as if they were penetrating into the deeper layers of the colon wall. A CT scan didn't show any thickening or inflammation of her small intestine. She also had some anal skin tags, which were contributing to her anal bleeding and discomfort. Because it was hard to determine whether Jennifer had ulcerative colitis or Crohn's disease limited to the colon, she was diagnosed with indeterminate colitis. The fact that the inflammation was located throughout her colon and no areas appeared normal suggested ulcerative colitis. But the deeper ulcers and the relative normal appearance of the rectum suggested Crohn's disease.

Because ulcerative colitis is confined to the colon, it stands to reason that inflammation found in the small intestine (ileum) must be Crohn's disease. However, as we discussed earlier, inflammation in the colon from ulcerative colitis can be so bad that it causes the valve that seals off the small intestine from the colon to also become inflamed, and some of the inflammation within the colon can "backwash" a few inches into the ileum. This inflammation isn't the same as the inflammation of Crohn's disease.

Some health care providers use specific protein markers in the blood to try to distinguish between the two conditions. People with colitis (either ulcerative colitis or Crohn's colitis) are more likely to have the protein p-ANCA in their blood than the rest of the population. ASCA, another marker, is more common in people with Crohn's disease, regardless of where their disease is located. There are even more specific proteins used to separate ulcerative colitis from Crohn's disease, but none of them are useful for making a diagnosis without other testing, such as endoscopy with biopsy.

MICROSCOPIC OR LYMPHOCYTIC COLITIS

Microscopic colitis is considered an inflammatory bowel disease because it involves inflammation of the colon lining. This condition, however, doesn't cause the ulceration seen in ulcerative colitis. It's called microscopic colitis because it can only be seen under a microscope. When a person with microscopic colitis has a colonoscopy, the lining appears totally typical. It's only when biopsy tissue samples are examined under a microscope that inflammation is seen.

At age 60, Mary Jane's life has been turned upside down by six months of bad diarrhea. She's going to the bathroom as much as 12 times a day and waking up at night to use the toilet as well. She hasn't seen any blood or lost any weight, although she can't understand why not, considering all the diarrhea. Her primary doctor suggested that she increase her fiber intake to bulk up her stools, which didn't help at all. A colonoscopy by a local surgeon found no evidence of active inflammation and no tumors or polyps. She was told it was "all in her head" and to take Imodium as needed. Unsatisfied, Mary Jane sought out another opinion. A second examination of her colon was normal, but when biopsies taken during the procedure were examined under a microscope, they revealed that Mary Jane had chronic inflammation typical of microscopic colitis. Ten days after receiving appropriate anti-inflammatory medication, she was back to having solid stools, and her life returned to normal.

The condition is also called lymphocytic colitis because certain white blood cells called lymphocytes cause the inflammation. In some patients, there's an increased layer of collagen found on biopsy.

Microscopic colitis mainly affects women. It may be an allergic-type reaction to a medicine, or it can happen for reasons that are unclear. Certain medications, such as nonsteroidal anti-inflammatory drugs like ibuprofen and acid-reducing medications like proton pump inhibitors and high blood pressure medicines, are associated with this condition. It's helpful, of course, if you can identify which medication is responsible.

Microscopic colitis causes watery diarrhea, sometimes up to 15 to 20 stools per day. There's no blood because there's no ulceration of the intestine lining. Usually there's no weight loss either, and as it was for Mary Jane, getting a correct diagnosis can take a while.

Some people respond to medications that relieve diarrhea. Others need medications that treat ulcerative colitis to get their inflammation under control. This type of colitis may disappear completely in some people.

COLLAGENOUS COLITIS

Collagenous colitis is another form of microscopic colitis. One of the important parts of the bowel wall, which gives it structure and strength, is the layer of collagen. Collagen, a protein known for its stretchiness, is found in joints, skin and other tissues.

For some reason, possibly an inflammatory process, this collagen layer overgrows and thickens in some people. When the collagen layer becomes too thick, it prevents water from reentering the colon wall, which is the main function of the colon. Unabsorbed water leads to watery diarrhea. Because there's no ulceration, there's no blood in the stool.

Women are more likely to have this condition. On visual examination, the lining of the colon appears typical. A diagnosis can only be made by examining biopsy samples under a microscope for a thickened collagen layer.

Pepto Bismol helps a small number of people, and others respond to common antidiarrheal medicines. For those who don't respond, anti-inflammatory medications used to treat ulcerative colitis are often prescribed.

Self-management:
It's your IBD

How IBD affects you is an individual matter. A major theme in this book is that one size doesn't fit all, so there's no single recipe for how to manage the disease. Think of IBD management as an ongoing discussion between you and your health care team. They make treatment recommendations, and you provide feedback on what worked and what didn't. Together, you identify ongoing challenges, set goals and discuss what to do next.

Management of the disease is truly a team effort, and your active involvement is a necessity. Medical providers are available to help you. Their support can help you avoid using your illness as an excuse to give up or drop out of life.

There's no single way to go about managing your IBD, but it's important to start

somewhere. Some important milestones, such as diagnosis and worsening of symptoms, require active medical management. This chapter outlines the kinds of management decisions that specialists generally discuss with their patients at each important milestone in their disease.

In initial meetings with an individual who has IBD, specialists usually have three types of plans in mind — immediate, short term and long term. The emphasis will be different for a person who's just been diagnosed than for an individual who's had IBD for some time and is experiencing a flare. What doctors generally want to do right away is deal with the one or two major symptoms that an individual is experiencing — often pain and diarrhea.

IMMEDIATE PLAN

Let's assume that you've just been diagnosed and you're at your doctor's office for a discussion about your test results. The first thing to determine is: Do you need to be in the hospital for treatment, or are you stable enough to go home with a treatment plan and care for yourself? To make this decision, we discuss the level of inflammation tests revealed and the location of the inflammation. This gives us an idea of how much damage has occurred, and it helps you to understand why you're having specific symptoms.

Whether you're in a hospital or you return home, the next part of the immediate plan centers on medication. Some medications suppress the inflammation and help treat symptoms, while others do just one or the other. If you're hospitalized, treatment generally includes intravenous medications such as steroids, antibiotics and fluids.

We know someone is stable enough to go home when they're able to take in adequate fluids and calories to sustain themselves, and bleeding and diarrhea are a fraction of what they were, though perhaps not gone.

Whenever you begin a new medication, it's important to follow up with your doctor within two weeks to discuss the results. It could be a phone call or message through the patient portal in your online medical account. Follow-up is the only way to know whether the treatment plan is working and you're tolerating the medication as prescribed.

Medication	Action	Used for
Steroids	Potent anti-inflammatory	IBD
Antibiotics	Anti-infection	Crohn's disease involving the anal area
5-ASA	Anti-inflammatory	Ulcerative colitis and some patients with Crohn's colitis
Immunomodulators	Anti-inflammatory	IBD
Biologics	Anti-inflammatory	IBD
Small molecules	Anti-inflammatory	Ulcerative colitis

This table lists the main categories of medications used to treat IBD. Each medication is discussed in detail in Chapter 6.

Kevin wasn't feeling well when he arrived at the hospital emergency room after three days of worsening abdominal pain, fever, nausea and vomiting. He had been to a friend's cookout a few days earlier and assumed he had food poisoning. A CT scan revealed a large abscess in his lower right side and a long segment of inflamed bowel. He quickly underwent surgery in which the surgeon drained the abscess, removed a piece of inflamed bowel and sewed Kevin back together with a bag to collect stool — a temporary ileostomy. The ileostomy was reversed eight weeks later.

There are several reasons why a plan may not work:

- The medication may not be strong enough for your level of disease activity. It's preferable to start with a medication that has limited side effects and hope that it will be enough to manage the inflammation.
- Your disease may be more active than expected. Patients sometimes minimize their symptoms so as to not appear to be a "wimp," in which case the chosen therapy may not be effective.
- You may be having side effects that keep you from taking the amount of medication you need.
- Not enough time has passed for you to experience the full benefits of the medication.
- A confounding factor is interfering with expected results, such as an ongoing or overlapping infection or a second condition, such as irritable bowel syndrome.

If you're allergic to the medication or dealing with a bad side effect, or if the medication is simply too expensive, we want to discuss this soon after you start the medication. This is the time for complete honesty with your health care provider about how you're doing.

Other urgent matters also may be part of the immediate plan. For someone diagnosed with Crohn's disease and a fistula, for example, surgery to repair the fistula may be needed. After a surgical procedure, follow-up exams to assess how well the wound is closing are scheduled, and you'll receive information on what you need to do to keep it closed.

SHORT-TERM PLAN

The two weeks between receiving a new prescription or starting a new treatment approach and seeing your doctor on a return visit to evaluate progress marks the transition from your immediate plan to your short-term plan.

A short-term plan may be as simple as continuing with your current medication regimen or increasing the dose if you're tolerating it but not having the kind of response expected. Your doctor may recommend a different or additional medication to achieve the desired re-

Kathy, who is 35, has Crohn's disease. She smokes cigarettes and, because she travels frequently for work, eats out often. She met with a doctor, complaining of cramping and bloating, and said she sometimes noticed undigested food in her stools. A colonoscopy didn't show any active disease. However, Kathy met with a dietitian, who taught her how to make better food choices when traveling. The next time she met with her doctor, her cramping and bloating had improved. Kathy was used to eating whenever was convenient, but now she avoids certain foods, like caffeine and tacos with refried beans, after 4:00 p.m.

sponse. You may need to taper the dose of a short-term medication (such as steroids) if the medication has produced the intended effect or if side effects are keeping you from taking as much as you really need (as might happen with the medication sulfasalazine).

If your medications are working as intended, then your short-term plan may involve testing. Your provider may want to evaluate your nutrition and bone health with tests that aren't generally done when making an IBD diagnosis. This kind of information might identify ways to improve your long-term health with different food choices or supplements and indicate whether visiting a dietitian would be helpful.

Now is also a good time to get you up to date on vaccinations, especially if you're taking medications that suppress your immune system. Before starting an immunosuppressant or immunomodulator, your doctor will want to check that you're current on all of your vaccines, including the COVID-19, human papillomavirus (HPV), pneumonia, influenza, hepatitis and shingles vaccines.

Information overload

There's a lot to know about living with IBD. And doctors and researchers learn something new every few months about treating Crohn's disease and ulcerative colitis. When first diagnosed, if you're presented with too much information at once, it can feel overwhelming. Plus, there's only so much you can take in and use right away.

For those of you who've had the disease for some time, understand that because our knowledge is growing so rapidly, things you were taught years ago might no longer be correct!

Often the best approach is to learn what you need to know to deal with immediate issues and then take in additional information to suit your needs at your own speed. But always stay curious and remember that understanding and treatment of IBD continue to evolve.

If you're looking for additional information, there are high-quality, reliable sources you can turn to when you're ready (see page 183). They include the

Crohn's & Colitis Foundation; the National Institutes of Health; and various universities, gastroenterology practices and pharmaceutical companies. All sources vary in their biases and their ability to stay up to date, so discuss the information, particularly concerning medications, with your health care provider. This is part of the ongoing conversation of living with IBD.

Self-awareness tools

You might consider keeping a diary of your symptoms that includes when and what you eat, your activities, and, if you're a woman, your menstrual cycle. There are several good apps available on the market and through organizations like the Crohn's & Colitis Foundation to help track symptoms, medications and your health history.

The information you gather can provide you and your doctor with valuable insight into your unique patterns and habits, which may help you self-manage your IBD. You might also keep a list of your test results on your cell phone or computer for easy reference, including dates of X-rays, endoscopic studies and your medications with dates and doses.

This may help you avoid undergoing tests that you've recently had or retaking medications that didn't work simply because you don't remember their names. And, of course, this is very valuable information if you see a new medical provider.

Goals

Another component of a short-term plan is to discuss realistic timelines as to when you should begin to see improvement from your therapy. Involving loved ones at this time can be important so that they can learn early in the disease process as

SAMPLE SYMPTOM DIARY

Date	Symptom	Activity before symptom	Action taken
June 21	Diarrhea	Ate at local diner	Took Imodium
July 3	Abdominal pain	Ate at picnic	Lay down

A symptom diary doesn't have to be fancy or detailed. The goal is to log symptoms, activities surrounding their development and steps taken to control them, to see if any type of pattern emerges.

Mark, an auto repair shop manager recently diagnosed with ulcerative colitis, was having 10 to 12 bloody bowel movements per day and rapidly began to lose weight. When diagnosed, he was hospitalized and treated with intravenous steroids. He was discharged from the hospital on oral steroids and later started on a biologic medication, but he never really got better. Mark continued to have multiple bloody stools every day and kept losing weight. When he went to get a second opinion, he had lost 20% of his original body weight and could hardly walk on his own power. He was anemic, malnourished and miserable. Unfortunately, there was little that medication could do to save Mark's badly inflamed colon, and doctors recommended surgery to remove it.

well. We encourage patients to bring along a spouse, friend or relative to the first few appointments.

The medications chapter (Chapter 6) describes in detail most of the medications currently in use to treat Crohn's disease and ulcerative colitis, how they work and when you may begin to see improvements. But medications do have their limitations, and in some cases, a short-term plan may include surgery.

Surgery can be a scary proposition, but your disease may be more aggressive than you or your health care provider realized. Some people do poorly, and can even die, if they delay surgery. As part of the team approach to managing your disease, it's important that you discuss openly any fears about surgery.

Other issues

As you begin to feel better, your short-term plan may expand to include lifestyle and quality-of-life issues. This is the time to discuss appropriate changes in how you eat, your work or school schedule and issues that may be on your mind regarding intimacy, family planning and all the what-ifs.

By understanding where you are in your life and issues of immediate concern, your doctor can help you to move forward. This also may be a good time to discuss certain overarching issues as well as make decisions regarding the appropriateness of medications and timing of follow-up appointments.

It's also time to visit your primary care provider and discuss your IBD diagnosis and treatment plan. Not every health issue you have will be IBD related, but it's important that your primary care provider be aware of all aspects of your disease.

You need both kinds of medical care — specialty care from a gastroenterologist and general care from a primary care provider.

LONG-TERM PLAN

Once you and your doctor have decided on the best therapy to manage your condition and the goals for your treatment, the long-term plan kicks in. This phase of your care is all about maintaining your remission, preventing flares and caring for your overall general health. Your health care team will work with you to formulate a health maintenance plan to maximize your quality of life.

Quality-of-life issues involve your goals, such as raising a family, finishing school, working and having personal relationships. Over time, quality-of-life issues change, as do personal dynamics, and it's important to recognize the ways in which your quality of life affects your health.

The information in the rest of this book will help you really understand what "self-management" of your disease means. Education will enable you to have meaningful discussions with your health care providers about what you're experiencing and help you identify and state your preferences in terms of immediate, short-term and long-term care.

HEALTH CARE TEAM

Having a team of medical professionals that you can turn to when you have questions or concerns can help you live well with a chronic disease. Your team should include a primary care doctor to oversee your general health and a gastroenterologist who specializes in IBD. In addition to these two individuals, your team may include a nurse practitioner (NP) or physician assistant (PA); the NPs and PAs in your gastroenterologist's office will be specially trained in GI issues.

We urge you to find health care professionals with whom you can have a helpful, informative conversation. Look for providers who are both good listeners and good teachers. Because you have IBD, there's a good chance that you'll eventually need to discuss private and often embarrassing things. If you feel more comfortable talking to either a woman or a man, then actively seek the right person to help you manage your care.

Primary care physician

Understandably, your IBD likely demands your full attention, but it's important to attend to your overall health and not focus only on your IBD. A primary care physician can look beyond your IBD at other health issues. Find a physician you feel comfortable with who'll take a holistic approach to your general health. This need becomes even more important as you get older and other health problems develop.

Remember, you're a product of your genes. If your family has a history of a specific disease, you may have inherited that risk, and it's important that you take steps to minimize it. In addition, your IBD treatment may increase your risk of other diseases. If you take steroids, for example, you may be at increased risk of diabetes and high blood pressure, so it's important to monitor your blood sugar (glucose) and blood pressure at age-appropriate times.

Your primary care physician may be a general practitioner or an internist. Both are medical doctors with training in all fields of medicine. He or she may be joined by a nurse practitioner or physician assistant, who also may be part of your health care team.

Your primary care physician may have been the individual who helped you get your IBD diagnosed and may be very helpful in your ongoing care. In some areas of the country, internists provide the bulk of the care for people with IBD and may refer you to a GI specialist only when your condition is complicated or specialized tests are needed.

Many people with IBD mistakenly believe that they shouldn't receive any vaccines. This isn't true. The vaccines that some people with IBD must avoid are those made up of live viruses, such as the polio, yellow fever and chickenpox vaccines, and the intranasal influenza (flu) vaccine. If any of these are needed, they should be given prior to any initiation of steroids, immunosuppressants or biologics. Once you're on these medications, your immune system may not fully respond to a vaccine, so it won't offer you as much protection from those diseases.

Vaccines against COVID-19, pneumonia, influenza, tetanus, hepatitis and shingles are still effective and safe and important to protect your health. These vaccines are all inactive and therefore can be

PREVENTIVE HEALTH CARE MEASURES

Colonoscopy
- Postoperative
- Surveillance for cancer and precancerous changes

Laboratory exams
- 25-hydroxyvitamin D
- B12/folate/iron
- CBC
- CMP
- CRP
- Lipids/glucose
- Liver enzymes

Radiology
- DEXA (dual-energy X-ray absorptiometry) scan
- Mammogram

Regular exams
- Breast/Pap test
- Prostate
- Blood pressure
- Ophthalmologic
- Skin cancer
- Tuberculosis (TB) test

Vaccinations
- COVID-19
- Hepatitis A
- Hepatitis B
- Human papillomavirus
- Influenza
- Mumps, measles, rubella
- Pneumococcal
- Shingles
- Td/Tdap (tetanus)
- Varicella

administered to all individuals, even people who are taking immunosuppressive medications. Some vaccines, such as the pneumococcal pneumonia and shingles vaccines, are given at an early age in people with IBD.

Doctors and researchers have learned much more about vaccines against COVID-19 since the onset of the pandemic. The Centers for Disease Control and Prevention (CDC) recommends that all people with IBD who are eligible should get vaccinated. COVID-19 vaccines are effective in people with IBD and aren't associated with worsening disease activity.

Contracting an infection such as COVID-19, pneumonia, influenza, tetanus, hepatitis or shingles could lead to a hospital admission that would require stopping your medications and lead to a relapse of your IBD symptoms.

Gastroenterologist

A gastroenterologist is a physician with an additional three to four years of training in the field of gastroenterology and hepatology. Our specialty is known affectionately as "guts and butts," so it includes diseases of the esophagus, stomach, liver, gallbladder, pancreas, small intestine and large intestine (colon and rectum).

Gastroenterologists aren't surgeons, but they do perform procedures such as colonoscopies. Surgeons perform operations such as removing the gallbladder or draining abscesses. Not all gastroenterologists have a special interest in IBD; we encourage you to find one who does.

Some gastroenterologists are particularly busy performing procedures, so the bulk of your regular care may be provided by a specially trained NP or PA who's part of your health care team. This person will oversee your follow-up appointments, consulting with your gastroenterologist.

NPs and PAs write prescriptions, order tests, offer referrals, and have their own office schedules. In locations where there are only a few gastroenterologists, NPs and PAs perform flexible sigmoidoscopies. They don't perform colonoscopies or other complex procedures.

In general, NPs and PAs often have more time to educate patients and may be more knowledgeable about living with IBD and the newest medications than many physicians.

GI specialty center

Some people wonder if they should be cared for at medical centers with a special focus on IBD. There are different levels of specialty, even within IBD. Centers that see more than just a few people with IBD per week tend to be the places that run clinical trials, offer the most up-to-date therapies and have the most experience with complicated cases. Such centers are also a good resource for second opinions, and staff can work with your local gastroenterologist to co-manage your condition.

A speciality center isn't for everyone. It's understood that visiting a specialty center may require you to travel if you don't live near such a facility. Some people also feel overwhelmed in the setting of a large institution and prefer a small office and seeing just one physician instead of several. In either situation, a virtual consultation with an IBD expert may be an option. Do what works best for you and your circumstances.

Surgeons

Surgeons perform operations as well as procedures such as colonoscopies. Individuals with ulcerative colitis who need to have a J-pouch procedure, for example, will see a surgeon. Because surgeons don't have specific training in the medical aspects of IBD, they are your go-to professional when you need surgery but are generally not the best person for your general and IBD care.

Hospitalists

Some medical practices have doctors who specialize in the care of hospitalized patients. Hospitalists may make decisions regarding your care when you're hospitalized with an IBD flare. Hospitalists generally work in conjunction with your health care provider. They typically don't play a role in your care once you're discharged from the hospital, though you may develop a strong bond with a hospitalist while you're going through some of the toughest days of living with IBD.

GETTING THE MOST FROM YOUR VISITS

When you see your doctor for a scheduled appointment, consider following these suggestions to make the most of that time:

- Have an agenda with a list of issues or topics you want to discuss in order of priority — in case you don't get to all of them during your visit.
- Bring someone else with you, or record your conversations or take notes, so that you don't forget valuable information after you leave the office.
- Be realistic in your expectations. Your health care provider doesn't have unlimited time to spend with you. Your appointment may run anywhere from 15 to 60 minutes.
- Ask how you can be proactive in managing your IBD. Your efforts are likely to pay off and may make future visits positive experiences.
- Request copies of your test results after each visit. Keeping records makes it easier to track your condition and to share your information with new health care providers. You also may be able to access this information from your online electronic medical record.

6

Medications for IBD

IBD isn't curable, but there are ways to manage the disease, and that includes use of medication. Medications help control inflammation, alleviate symptoms, and prevent long-term consequences. Medications are very important to managing IBD, but they can't replace good lifestyle habits, and they need to be taken in the appropriate manner to be effective.

Why might your doctor prescribe medication? Some drugs help control symptoms, such as antidiarrheals and pain medications. Others, such as steroids, control inflammation. Therapies such as azathioprine and biologics help heal your intestinal lining.

The table on pages 74–81 summarizes common therapies used to treat IBD.

Additional medications may be available through clinical trials. In a clinical trial, also called a clinical study, drugs are tested in a controlled manner to determine their effectiveness compared with other medications or compared to not taking any medication. Clinical trials are also used to determine the safety and potential side effects of a medication.

Many of the medications discussed in this chapter have been tested in clinical trials and approved by the Food and Drug Administration (FDA) for the treatment of ulcerative colitis and Crohn's disease.

Some medications used to treat IBD aren't FDA approved, but they've been shown to be effective in individuals with Crohn's disease or ulcerative colitis.

Seventeen-year-old Sharon was diagnosed with Crohn's disease after a trip to the hospital emergency department and the results of a CT scan. She was prescribed prednisone, and within a day her pain was significantly improved, and she was able to eat. Her diarrhea also got better within a couple more days. However, she developed acne and was unable to sleep as a result of feeling so wired. Tad also received prednisone after his diagnosis. However, his symptoms didn't get better. That's because Tad's symptoms were the result of a narrowed, scarred section of bowel without any active inflammation.

ANTI-INFLAMMATORY MEDICATIONS

Anti-inflammatory drugs are often the first step in the treatment of inflammatory bowel disease. Anti-inflammatory drugs include steroid medications and drugs known as aminosalicylates.

Steroids

Steroids, also referred to as corticosteroids, have been the cornerstone of medical treatment for active IBD since the 1950s. They're inexpensive, work quickly, and can be given orally, intravenously or rectally as suppositories. If your symptoms are severe, steroids can often relieve them quickly. Steroids work by essentially shutting down your entire immune system, which helps control the inflammatory reaction in the GI tract. Although this is an effective strategy for IBD symptoms, it comes with a big price in terms of side effects.

Whether you have ulcerative colitis or Crohn's disease, steroid use requires careful consideration. Using steroids for a lengthy period can lead to significant side effects. So, when you and your doctor decide on a course of steroids, there should be a clear plan for going off the medication — an exit strategy. It's important to avoid the medications if you have osteoporosis, an infection, uncontrolled diabetes or a history of significant psychiatric side effects when taking steroids, such as psychosis or suicidal thoughts.

The most common form of oral steroids for adults is prednisone and for children under age 16, methylprednisolone. A typical starting dose is 40 milligrams per day, given either once a day or, more likely, in divided doses. Divided doses allow for a more even level of steroid availability throughout the day, as opposed to a lot of medicine in the morning and none by the end of the day. Steroids should always be taken with food to minimize the potential for an upset stomach.

Steroids are most often prescribed when an individual is hospitalized for IBD. In the hospital, intravenous (IV) doses are

THE SAME, BUT DIFFERENT

There's one steroid that can help mild to moderate Crohn's disease without the typical steroid side effects. Budesonide (Entocort EC) may work as well as prednisone for Crohn's disease located in the terminal ileum and right side of the colon.

Unlike regular prednisone, budesonide doesn't circulate as long in the bloodstream. After taking the medication by mouth, it's absorbed in the last part of the small intestine and in parts of the colon. The liver then takes close to 90% of the drug out of action. This makes it an effective locally acting steroid. It's not as effective when Crohn's disease is spread over a larger area of the GI tract or during periods of very active inflammation. If you find budesonide helpful, you might use it for several months before needing to be weaned off.

Another form of budesonide called budesonide MMX (UCERIS) has been shown to be effective in mild to moderate ulcerative colitis.

generally administered until disease activity is controlled, and then the switch is made to oral steroid medications. Some people have problems after they're discharged from the hospital if they were transitioned too quickly from the intravenous to the oral steroids. Therefore, before leaving the hospital, it's important to know you are tolerating the medication and can stay well on oral therapy.

Side effects of steroid use can include weight gain, mood swings, acne, hair loss, problems with blood flow to the larger joints, increased risk for infections, increased appetite and energy level, and higher blood sugar (glucose) levels.

Having increased energy may sound positive, but this may come in the form of anxiety and jitteriness, along with insomnia. Regarding mental health, steroid use tends to make the highs higher and the lows lower. So a good mood can feel euphoric, and if you're sad, you may be tearful and even depressed.

When steroids are used long term (longer than six weeks), side effects may include thinning of the skin, easy bruising, osteoporosis, steroid-induced diabetes, high blood pressure and cataracts. Individuals on steroids are more at risk for complications when they're in accidents, have surgery or get another illness.

Because your body's adrenal glands naturally make about 5 to 7 milligrams of prednisone a day, taking steroids sends a message to the glands to shut down because they aren't needed. That's why it's important to wean yourself off steroids slowly and carefully. Tapering allows your body to determine it has to trigger the adrenal glands to start making prednisone again. Patients who are weaned too quickly can go through withdrawal, which is characterized by light-headedness, weakness, headache, joint pains and sometimes fainting and loss of consciousness.

Even years down the road, the effects of steroids can remain with you. If you take steroids for a prolonged period, thin, fragile veins (varicose veins), cataracts, and diabetes are a few conditions that can develop long after the medications are stopped. Because everyone has a different threshold for sensitivity to steroids, the definition of "a long period" varies. But if you've been treated with 10 milligrams or more for more than four months, you could experience long-term effects.

Steroids are also available in the form of an enema. Side effects with enemas aren't as frequent as with oral steroids, but because the medication is still absorbed into the bloodstream, steroids delivered via enema should be limited to no longer than about 12 weeks. Alternatives to steroid enemas are also available.

As doctors learn more about alternatives to steroids, they're finding that use of steroid medications is often associated with the worst outcome in patients. Whenever possible, doctors will try to avoid steroids and use alternative medications. However, because steroids can provide quick relief of symptoms, they're considered a "necessary evil" and are still prescribed.

Aminosalicylates

This class of drugs works within the lining of the gut. Because the medications don't affect the immune system like steroids, aminosalicylates are considered the safest IBD medications.

The active ingredient of these anti-inflammatory drugs is 5-aminosalicylic acid (5-ASA). Although related to aspirin

When 31-year-old Michael was diagnosed with ulcerative colitis, he was started on a 5-ASA drug that he took twice a day. He noticed a difference in his symptoms within two weeks. By eight weeks, they had completely resolved. Joann's ulcerative colitis symptoms were a little more severe than Michael's. She was having as many as eight stools each day and even some in the middle of the night. She required a higher dose of 5-ASA for her more moderately active disease. Her symptoms improved after about two weeks, but it took at least 10 weeks for her diarrhea to stop.

(salicylic acid) and other pain relievers, aminosalicylates are very distant relatives. They use completely different methods for treating inflammation.

There are different forms of 5-ASA, namely, mesalamine, balsalazide, olsalazine and sulfasalazine. All work by "mopping up" the proteins in the lining of the gut that cause inflammation. The medications don't inhibit the proteins from being made, but they stop them from being able to work. Think of 5-ASAs as brooms that sweep dirt off the floor. The broom doesn't stop the dirt from collecting; it just cleans it up after the fact.

5-ASAs are FDA-approved to treat active disease and maintain remission for ulcerative colitis. The medications are effective and associated with few side effects. In fact, in some studies, long-term use has been associated with a decreased risk of cancer. Some people with Crohn's disease are also prescribed 5-ASAs, but data suggest they're not effective unless the disease is confined to the colon or is in the small intestine and mild.

With this class of drugs, the thinking is "more can be better." Some people with more aggressive disease may need up to 4.8 grams daily, whereas others only need half that much. There's no increase in side effects with an increased dose, so if your disease requires additional medication to relieve your symptoms, you can use more.

The exception to this approach is sulfasalazine, which does cause an increase in side effects the more you take. Sulfasalazine is a very effective drug that also helps with joint pain (see Chapter 7 for more about IBD-associated joint pain). Many people, however, are intolerant to or allergic to the sulfa in this medication, which is why the sulfa-free agents were developed.

All aminosalicylates can be taken twice daily, or only once a day if that's all you need. It was once recommended they be taken three or four times a day, but with decades of use and further study, we've found that's not necessary. There are some subtle differences between the drugs, just like differences between brands of peanut butter or toothpaste. All the agents in this class of drugs essentially work the same, so it's a matter of preference in terms of capsules or pills, amount of medicine per unit and cost.

Occasionally, patients experience worsening symptoms on 5-ASAs, usually within a few days of starting them. If your diarrhea and bleeding worsen when taking a 5-ASA medication, it may be an indication of an allergic-type reaction to the medicine. The same thing will happen with any of the other medications in this class, so it doesn't help to switch from one to another. You and your doctor will need to find an alternative drug to treat your disease.

For people who tolerate 5-ASA medications and experience a benefit, there are some rare side effects to watch for. They include hair loss, headache, inflammation of the lining of the lungs or heart, inflammation of the pancreas and kidney damage. Sulfasalazine, in particular, can damage bone marrow. So, taking these medications requires some additional blood monitoring to ensure your safety.

IMMUNOMODULATORS

Immunomodulators work by modifying immune system activity, decreasing the body's inflammatory response. Immunomodulators were originally developed to treat leukemia and are most often used in individuals receiving organ transplants to prevent rejection of the new organ and in individuals with autoimmune diseases, such as rheumatoid arthritis.

At much lower doses, they help control the part of the immune system responsible for uncontrolled inflammatory responses, such as those associated with IBD. There are several medications used to treat Crohn's disease and ulcerative colitis that fall into this category.

6-mercaptopurine and azathioprine

These immunomodulators are commonly used to treat ulcerative colitis and both the inflammatory and the fistulizing types of Crohn's disease. Because they suppress the actions of just one part of the immune system rather than the entire immune system, as do steroids, they're typically safer than steroids. Immunomodulators can help individuals avoid or stop using steroids. For this reason, they're often referred to as steroid-sparing drugs.

There are some important things to know about immunomodulators for IBD management. First, although they're effective, it may take anywhere from three to six months of use before you notice their full benefit. Also, since the introduction of biologic medications, immunomodulators are often used in combination with biologics to prevent an antibody response to biologic therapy.

Also, this class of medications has the potential for short- and long-term side effects. Therefore, it's important that you and your doctor work together to ensure proper use and monitoring. You might view taking these medications as similar to receiving the keys to a fancy sports car. Put them in the hands of a novice 16-year-old driver and there's likely to be trouble,

Sharon experienced relief of her severe Crohn's symptoms after being treated with steroids to control the inflammation. She then needed something to manage her disease instead of the steroids. Her doctor recommended an immunomodulator. As she tapered off the steroids, she began taking the new medication, which built up slowly in her system. Within three months of starting the medication, Sharon was off steroids and feeling well.

but in the right hands, a high-performance machine can deliver a safe experience.

Short-term side effects of the drugs, sometimes called allergies, include:
- Fever, as high as 103 F.
- Rash.
- Back pain.
- Joint pain.
- Pancreatitis (inflammation of the pancreas).

Side effects occur in the first three to four weeks of use in about 7% to 10% of individuals who take the drugs. If you experience any of these reactions, you shouldn't remain on this type of medication. However, if mild nausea is your only symptom, taking the medications at night or with food can often alleviate the nausea.

Another common side effect happens when the drug does its job too well and decreases your white blood cell count, making you susceptible to infections and illness. A decreased white blood cell count is entirely reversible when the medication is stopped. Most often, a doctor will restart it at a lower dose. Because you don't experience symptoms from a decreased white blood cell count, it's important that you undergo regular blood tests.

There are specific tests called TMPT and NUDT15 that help doctors know how efficiently you're able to metabolize azathioprine and 6-mercaptopurine (6-MP). (Azathioprine is broken down by the body and turned into 6-MP, so they are essentially the same drug.) In fact, the TMPT and NUDT15 enzyme tests are generally done prior to deciding on a medication dose because these tests can help predict your risk for a decreased white blood cell count. Other tests may also be performed in certain individuals to determine the safety of using azathioprine or 6-MP.

Immunomodulators may cause slight liver damage, which is also monitored with blood tests. If your liver becomes damaged, this is reversible by stopping the drug or decreasing the dosage.

Perhaps the most frightening long-term effect of the drug is the association of immunomodulators with the development of cancer of the lymph nodes (lymphoma). Here are two key points to keep in mind about this:
- The overall risk is still very small.
- Alternatives to immunomodulator use — experiencing active disease or taking steroids — are associated with increased risks, including death. Taking an immunomodulator, meanwhile, may actually lower your risk of serious complications.

Methotrexate

Another commonly used immunomodulator is methotrexate. This drug was adopted as a treatment for Crohn's disease from rheumatologists, who use it to treat rheumatoid arthritis. In addition to treating inflammation, it's particularly helpful for relieving painful, swollen joints. Although available in both pill and shot form, the medication is usually given by injection because it isn't easily absorbed by an inflamed GI tract. Methotrexate is typically faster acting than 6-MP or azathioprine, is inexpensive, and is taken just once a week by self-injection.

On the downside, a methotrexate shot can cause flulike symptoms that can last 24 hours. The drug competes with the body for folic acid, so you need to take folic acid supplements daily. As with the other immunomodulators, you'll need blood tests to monitor liver function and your white blood cell count.

There isn't as high a risk of lymphoma with this medication, but it can increase your risk of lung damage with long-term use. A detailed discussion with your doctor is important if you have other health issues that also put you at risk for liver damage, such as diabetes, obesity or excessive alcohol use. Overall, methotrexate is effective with proper monitoring.

Cyclosporine

Cyclosporine is used for severely active ulcerative colitis, fistulas and a skin condition associated with IBD called pyoderma gangrenosum (see Chapter 7). This antirejection medication, given to people who've received an organ transplant to prevent possible organ rejection, also appears to help people with IBD in certain situations.

Cyclosporine is given intravenously in the hospital, and it works over a matter of days. If you're not getting any benefit within three to four days, the medication should be stopped. Use of this medication

has declined since approval of the drug infliximab for moderate to severe ulcerative colitis. Although effective, cyclosporine can lead to blood, potassium and magnesium abnormalities, as well as high blood pressure and kidney damage. Because of these side effects, the medication should be used for short periods (three months or less). It's also given intravenously to treat fistulas and pyoderma gangrenosum.

Tacrolimus

Another immunomodulator, tacrolimus is particularly helpful for people with IBD who have fistulas that don't respond to other medications. Tacrolimus comes in pill form and as a cream for topical use. An unpopular side effect of the medication is diarrhea. This isn't very welcome among individuals who are already prone to or have diarrhea. If you take this medication, regular blood tests are important because kidney damage can occur when drug levels are too high.

BIOLOGICS

For individuals who can't tolerate or don't respond to an immunomodulator, the availability of biologic therapy has been revolutionary. The first biologic to become available was infliximab (Remicade), approved in 1998.

Biologics make up a new class of drug treatment. They aren't chemicals but natural sources, including proteins and other substances, that are grown in a special factory. In the case of IBD, biologics inhibit the activity of specific immune system proteins that are causing inflammation. One target is tumor necrosis factor (TNF), an inflammatory protein involved in a variety of medical conditions. Blocking its activity allows the body to heal.

Currently, biologics used to treat IBD are delivered via either intravenous or intramuscular injections. Because they're proteins, if they were given orally, stomach acid would break them down and render them inactive. The medications are made by replicating the exact original antibody protein over and over. Each biologic agent is patented; this is what makes these drugs so expensive and why there will never be generic versions.

Biologics work relatively quickly, and they can be used instead of steroids or to help you get off steroids. But you can't just take them as needed. With experience, doctors have come to understand that once you start taking one of these medications, you need to continue to use it. And once you stop using it, your body may form antibodies to the biologic agent that, via an allergic reaction, renders the medicine inactive.

Think of a biologic as similar to a relative who comes to stay with you for a while. At first you may not like the individual, but you gradually get used to the person's ways and routines. If the relative leaves for a while and then comes back, you remember why you didn't initially care for that person. Instead of gradually

getting used to the person one more time, you rally the person to leave again. That's how your body deals with biologics. For the medication to keep working, you need to stay on it. That's a big commitment, so doctors usually save biologics for people with more active, severe IBD.

Types of biologics

Infliximab (Remicade), which has been on the market for over 20 years, is given intravenously to treat inflammatory or fistulizing Crohn's disease and ulcerative colitis. It's engineered to be 75% human protein and 25% mouse protein. Since it was first approved, three more anti-TNF agents have become available.

Adalimumab (Humira) is an injectable biologic that treats active Crohn's disease and ulcerative colitis. It's made from 100% human protein. Certolizumab pegol (Cimzia) is also injectable and given monthly. It treats active Crohn's disease and is 100% human. Golimumab (Simponi), another injectable drug, is approved to treat ulcerative colitis.

Researchers used to think that it mattered how much of a biologic is non-human, but it turns out that because all of these proteins are foreign to your body, there's just as much chance of reacting to a medication that's part mouse as to one that's all human.

Some people prefer infliximab because it's given at an infusion center where health care professionals are available in case there are any problems during or

BIOSIMILARS

Biosimilar medications are similar to the biologic drugs that they're manufactured to imitate, but their structures aren't quite the same.

Recently, a biosimilar to Remicade was approved. There are now several approved biosimilars for Remicade (Inflectra, Renflexis, Avsola). And it's expected that over the next several years there will be biosimilars for Humira as well. There's accumulating evidence that switching from Remicade to a biosimilar is safe, and doctors generally don't object to their patients making these switches or starting with a biosimilar.

after the infusion. This also offers the opportunity to socialize with others who have IBD and are receiving infusions that day. (We've had more than one romance develop among patients meeting regularly for infliximab infusions!) This time can also be a chance to catch up on reading or watch a movie.

Other people prefer the convenience of administering an adalimumab shot themselves every other week. Still others can't imagine giving themselves an injection — even though it's with a short, fine needle similar to an EpiPen — and they're more comfortable going to their doctor's office to receive an injection of certolizumab pegol each month or having a nurse come to their home.

Side effects

As noted earlier, biologics are antibodies, and your body can form its own antibody against an antibody. Yes, this is confusing.

What it means is that biologics may be associated with an allergic (hypersensitivity) reaction or a loss of response.

In the case of infliximab, an allergic response leads to hives, shortness of breath, wheezing, and sometimes fever and chills during the infusion and potentially lasting for a week after. Some people also develop bad joint pain and swelling, symptoms that are easy to mistake for the flu. Joint pain and swelling are different from an allergic reaction that may occur with initial use of a biologic. (In the latter instance, your body has an immediate reaction to the antibody by yet a different mechanism that doesn't require any prior exposure to the agent at all.)

Premedication with an antihistamine and Tylenol, plus a one-time shot of steroids, can often prevent a hypersensitivity reaction. Not everyone who receives infliximab is premedicated, but some physicians do follow such a protocol.

If you experience a reaction despite premedication, especially if it's quite severe, then you're considered allergic to that medication. You may be switched to another biologic, because being allergic to one biologic doesn't mean you'll have a similar reaction to the others. With the injectable biologics, allergic reactions — large hives, redness and swelling — can occur at the injection site.

Sometimes, rather than having an allergic reaction, your body develops antibodies that simply make the drug ineffective. Despite your infusion or injection, you don't feel like you've gotten any benefit. When this happens, your doctor might try increasing the dose or decreasing the time between doses. However, for some people, the medication stops working altogether. One way to avoid these possible reactions is to give the medications on a regular basis. If you take them irregularly, you're much more likely to develop an allergic or immune reaction. That is why it's so important to commit to a biologic once the decision has been made to use it.

Infliximab (Remicade), adalimumab (Humira), certolizumab pegol (Cimzia) and golimumab (Simponi) are all associated with an increased risk of infections because they act by deactivating tumor necrosis factor (TNF), an important immune system component that helps fight infection. Anti-TNF drugs increase the risk for infections from bacteria, viruses and certain kinds of fungi inhaled through the air. The medications can reactivate tuberculosis (TB) or hepatitis B if it's lying dormant in your body. Therefore, it's mandatory to undergo a TB test as well as a hepatitis B test before starting this therapy. While blood monitoring isn't required during biologic use, it's important to pay careful attention to new symptoms that might suggest an infection.

Another risk associated with biologics is lymphoma, which is cancer of the lymph nodes. Note the words *associated with* and not *caused by*. It's unclear why individuals using biologics — for any condition, not just IBD — appear to have a higher rate of certain types of lymphoma than people with the same disease who aren't taking biologics or people who are healthy and don't have IBD.

Researchers are following large registries of patients who are taking these medications to try to gain a better sense of what's being reported as well as changing trends. The risk of cancer of the lymph nodes (lymphoma) appears to be a risk with biologic medications. How much of a risk? If we agree that the risk in the healthy population of getting lymphoma is about 2 in 10,000, then use of a biologic doubles or triples the risk to about 4 to 6 people in 10,000.

Newer biologics

Vedolizumab (Entyvio) is a newer biologic. Unlike other drugs, it's not directed toward the TNF protein but to another protein that blocks cell movement and attachment to the lining of the gut. The medication is approved for use in moderate to severely active Crohn's disease and

Twenty-seven-year-old Renee has a history of Crohn's disease involving more than 70% of her small intestine. She was on steroids for years at a time and had to have a hip replacement due to bone damage from her prolonged exposure to the drugs. Because most of her bowel is involved in the disease, surgery isn't an option. Renee was on Remicade for years, then she stopped responding to it. She was switched to Humira, and then Cimzia, but lost response to those as well. She chose Entyvio and has been on it for close to a year now. She is doing well — well enough to get married!

ulcerative colitis. It also helps reduce use of steroids.

Because it only works on the lining of the gut, vedolizumab may only be prescribed by gastroenterologists and only in patients who haven't responded to or can't get off steroids.

Ustekinumab (Stelara) has been available as a treatment for psoriasis for several years and was recently approved as a medication for Crohn's disease and ulcerative colitis. Ustekinumab works on a different part of the immune system — not TNF. It's given as a one-time IV infusion, followed by shots every eight weeks.

Putting it all in perspective

After reading about biologics, perhaps the idea of using one sounds scary. Doctors typically don't view the medications that way. Biologics have provided hope to many individuals with very active Crohn's disease or ulcerative colitis who couldn't tolerate other medications or lost response to them. Each biologic

approved by the FDA has demonstrated an ability to decrease the risk of hospitalization, increase quality of life and ease the burden of living with IBD by reducing disease activity and lengthening the time between flares.

Studies show patients are often more willing to take risks than doctors if a therapy has a good chance of working, because the perceived benefit is higher than the perceived risk. Every treatment decision is a balancing act between benefit and risk, as are many decisions in life.

Think about something as simple as deciding to get in the car and drive to the grocery store. Does getting groceries outweigh the risk of getting harmed in a car accident? Until biologics came along, many people with IBD had to live with the downside of continuous steroid use; now, biologics have improved their quality of life.

SMALL MOLECULES

Small molecule medications, which also target immune system function, are a

Medication use is more common with age. That's why for older adults with IBD, it's especially important to make your doctor aware of all the medications that you take. Knowing each of the medications you use — prescription and nonprescription — will help your doctor determine if any of them could be negatively affecting your IBD.

For example, if you have arthritis, you may be taking a nonsteroidal anti-inflammatory drug (NSAID), which can cause a flare. Even over-the-counter NSAIDs can trigger a flare when added to prescription medications. Don't stop taking any medication prescribed by a health care provider, but make sure to review your medications with the doctor managing your IBD treatment.

Another issue when treating older adults is determining which medications to prescribe to treat IBD. With age, the body doesn't break down and use medications in the manner it once did. You may have become more sensitive to certain medications and need less, or you may not absorb the medication as well (or at all) and need more of or a different drug.

Some people take so many medications that it's almost impossible to predict the potential effects of various drugs.

Here's a short list of the known effects of IBD medications in older adults:
- Aminosalicylates are well tolerated.
- Azathioprine and 6-MP are also generally well tolerated, although given their slow onset of action, they aren't much use if you're acutely ill with IBD.

Also, the risk of infections such as shingles, as well as lymphoma and skin cancer, is higher in older adults.
- Topical medications, such as suppositories and enemas, may not be the best choices. It may be more difficult for older people with arthritis, for example, to self-administer rectal therapies.
- Corticosteroids have a higher risk of serious complications. Side effects include osteoporosis, cataracts, glaucoma, diabetes, psychosis, depression, infections, electrolyte abnormalities, congestive heart failure and high blood pressure. Some of these conditions, like drug-induced diabetes, will go away if you stop taking the steroids. Other conditions, like cataracts, require treatment and even surgery.
- Certain biologics are safer than others, and your doctor may choose a specific medication based on your age. Regardless of your age, however, biologics can be useful to control active inflammation and ultimately are safer than steroids.
- Small molecule medications haven't been adequately tested in older adults to fully understand their potential side effects. It is known that older people are at higher risk for eye issues, heart problems and shingles.

new class of medications that may be prescribed to treat ulcerative colitis.

Tofacitinib

Tofacitinib (Xeljanz) is a pill taken twice daily for moderate to severe ulcerative colitis. It works relatively quickly to provide relief of symptoms and, for the most part, is well tolerated. Tofacitinib is approved for individuals who don't respond to anti-TNF biologic medications.

A possible side effect of the medication is an increased chance of developing shingles. Getting vaccinated with the shingles vaccine SHINGRIX before starting Xeljanz is a good idea. In addition, the FDA recently issued a warning about tofacitinib, stating that preliminary studies show an increased risk of serious heart-related problems, blood clots and cancer from taking this drug.

If you're taking tofacitinib for ulcerative colitis, don't stop taking the medication without first talking with your doctor.

Ozanimod

Ozanimod (Zeposia) is another small molecule medication. First approved to treat relapsing forms of multiple sclerosis, it was approved to treat moderate to severe ulcerative colitis in 2021. The medication comes in pill form and is taken once daily. Because of potential side effects, you should be screened for specific heart and eye issues before taking the medication.

ANTIBIOTICS

Antibiotics are prescribed to fight infections that can develop in people with Crohn's disease, as well as abscesses and fistulas around the anal area.

An increasingly common infection among individuals with IBD is *Clostridioides difficile* infection. Some background here is helpful. Your digestive tract naturally contains many different bacteria, including a certain bacterium called *Clostridioides difficile* (*C. difficile* or *C. diff.*), which is normally present in a healthy gut.

When you take an antibiotic, it can wipe out certain kinds of bacteria, and sometimes *C. difficile* can multiply. This bacterium produces a toxin that, at high levels, causes inflammation. Overgrowth of *C. difficile* is common among residents of nursing homes and people who are hospitalized.

Unfortunately, with the high use of antibiotics in the general public, *C. difficile* strains are developing that are resistant to conventional treatment. People without any other risk factors are developing *C. difficile* infections, and individuals with IBD seem to be even more susceptible. The infection can result in flares, hospitalizations, and even death. It's diagnosed by testing stool for the presence of the toxin and treating the infection with the drug vancomycin or, in some cases, the antibiotic fidaxomicin.

C. difficile travels as spores, which can live outside the body and on surfaces for up to 60 days. The best way to prevent and control *C. difficile* is with vigorous handwashing and by cleaning surfaces that have been in contact with stool with a bleach-based solution.

In some people, *C. difficile* infection keeps coming back. These individuals usually need prolonged courses of antibiotics. A procedure called fecal

MEDICATIONS COMMONLY USED TO TREAT IBD INFLAMMATION

Name	Class	FDA IBD indication	Common uses
Prednisone, methylprednisolone, hydrocortisone	Systemic corticosteroid	None	Moderate to severe UC, CD
Budesonide (Entocort)	Local-acting corticosteroid	Mild to moderate CD of terminal ileum and colon	Ileocecal CD
Budesonide (UCERIS)	Local-acting corticosteroid	Mild to moderate UC	UC
Budesonide (UCERIS foam)	Topical/rectal steroid	Mild to moderate distal UC	Proctitis, active left-sided symptoms
Cortifoam, Cortenema, Proctofoam	Topical/rectal steroid	None	Proctitis, active left-sided symptoms
pH-controlled mesalamine (Asacol HD)	5-ASA	Mild to moderate UC	UC
Time-released mesalamine (Pentasa)	5-ASA	Mild to moderate UC	Small and large bowel CD, UC
MMX mesalamine (Lialda)	5-ASA	Mild to moderate UC	UC

microtbiota transfer (FMT) also has been successful in getting rid of the infection. For this procedure, stool from a healthy individual is processed and inserted into a patient with *C. difficile* via a colonoscope or by taking odorless and tasteless pills. Healthy bacteria quickly take up residence in their new environment.

Dosing	Common adverse events	Special considerations
1 to 2 mg/kg to a max of 40 to 60 mg orally per day	Weight gain, acne, mood changes, puffy face, increased appetite	Not for long-term use; patients doing well on steroids aren't in true remission; may affect growth in children
9 mg orally for 8 wks, 6 mg for 2 wks, then off	Same as prednisone but less frequent	Safer than prednisone but not for long-term use; also used for collagenous colitis, microscopic colitis
9 mg orally for 6 wks, 6 mg for 2 wks, then off	Same as prednisone but less frequent	Safer than prednisone but not for long-term use
Rectal application once to twice daily	Weight gain, headache	Some systemic absorption
Rectal application once to twice daily	Weight gain, headache	Some systemic absorption
2.4-4.8 g orally (800 mg tablets)	Headache, diarrhea, abdominal pain	3%-7% have worsening of colitis
2-4 g orally (250 mg or 500 mg capsules)	Headache, diarrhea, abdominal pain	3%-7% have worsening of colitis
2.4-4.8 g orally (1.2 g capsules)	Headache, diarrhea, abdominal pain	3%-7% have worsening of colitis

Name	Class	FDA IBD indication	Common uses	
Granular mesalamine (Apriso)	5-ASA	Maintenance of UC	UC	
Balsalazide (Giazo)	5-ASA	Mild to moderate UC	UC	
Olsalazine (Dipentum)	5-ASA	Maintenance of UC	UC	
Sulfasalazine (Azulfidine)	5-ASA	None	UC	
Mesalamine suppository (Canasa)	Topical 5-ASA	Active ulcerative proctitis	Proctitis	
Mesalamine enema (Rowasa)	Topical 5-ASA	Active mild to moderate distal UC, proctosigmoiditis or proctitis	Proctitis, left-sided colitis	
Azathioprine (Azasan, Imuran)	Immunomodulator	None	More commonly CD but also UC	
6-mercaptopurine (Purinethol)	Immunomodulator	None	More commonly CD but also UC	
Cyclosporine (Neoral, Sandimmune)	Immunomodulator	None	Severe UC and CD, fistulizing CD	
Methotrexate (Trexall)	Immunomodulator	None	CD	
Tacrolimus (Protopic)	Topical ointment	None	Cutaneous, perineal, perianal CD, pyoderma gangrenosum	
Tacrolimus (Prograf)	Immunomodulator	None	Moderate to severe UC and CD, fistulizing CD	

Dosing	Common adverse events	Special considerations
1.5 g orally (375 mg capsules)	Headache, diarrhea, abdominal pain	3%-7% have worsening of colitis
6.75 g orally (750 mg capsules)	Headache, diarrhea, abdominal pain	3%-7% have worsening of colitis
2-3 g orally (500 mg capsules)	Watery diarrhea	
3-6 g orally (500 mg capsules)	Rash, nausea, headache	Folic acid supplementation recommended
1,000 mg rectally once or twice daily (1,000 mg suppository)	Bloating, gas	Can be used in combination with oral 5-ASA
4 g per rectum at night (4 g enema)	Bloating, gas, incontinence	Often used in combination with oral 5-ASA
2-2.5 mg/kg body weight orally (50, 75, 100 mg)	Low blood counts, pancreatitis, rash, fevers	Regular blood counts essential for monitoring
1-1.5 mg/kg body weight orally (50 mg tablets)	Low blood counts, pancreatitis, rash, fevers	Regular blood counts essential for monitoring
2-4 mg/kg via IV, then 2x IV dose orally	Hypertension, headache, tremors, facial hair growth, low magnesium	Levels need to be monitored to avoid complications; Bactrim for prophylaxis of pneumonia
25 mg injection for 12 wks, then 15 mg maintenance	Mouth ulcers, liver damage, scarring of lungs	Folic acid supplementation recommended; absolutely not used in pregnancy
Strength 0.03%-0.1%, apply to affected area once to twice daily	Itching, burning of skin	Minimal absorption, but levels should be monitored initially
0.1-0.3 mg/kg dose orally twice daily	Nausea, heartburn, diarrhea, kidney damage	Levels must be monitored; risks may outweigh potential benefits

Name	Class	FDA IBD indication	Common uses	
Ciprofloxacin (Cipro)	Antibiotic	None	Fistulizing and colonic CD	
Metronidazole (Flagyl)	Antibiotic	None	Fistulizing and colonic CD	
Rifaximin (Xifaxan)	Antibiotic	None	Fistulizing and colonic CD	
Infliximab (Remicade) and infliximab biosimilars (Inflectra, Renflexis, Avsola)	Biologic agent (anti-TNF)	Inflammatory and fistulizing CD, UC	Moderate to severe CD and UC, pouchitis, joint and skin problems associated with IBD	
Adalimumab (Humira)	Biologic agent (anti-TNF)	Inflammatory CD, UC	Moderate to severe CD, UC	
Certolizumab pegol (Cimzia)	Biologic agent (anti-TNF)	Inflammatory CD	Moderate to severe CD	

Dosing	Common adverse events	Special considerations
500-1,000 mg orally daily	Rash, headache, diarrhea	Interacts with nutritional supplements
500-1,000 mg orally daily	Potential interaction with alcohol, metallic taste, nerve damage	Long-term use often limited by nerve damage; dose reduction may decrease risk
600-1,200 mg orally daily	Nausea, diarrhea, abdominal pain	Used for traveler's diarrhea and irritable bowel syndrome with diarrhea
5-10 mg/kg via IV induction at wks 0, 2, 6, then every 8 wks for maintenance	Infusion reactions, delayed hypersensitivity, upper respiratory infection (URI) symptoms, other infections	TB and hepatitis B tests must be performed prior to initiating since increased risk of TB and hepatitis B; possible to develop either intolerance or nonresponse over time
160 mg, 80 mg induction every other week, then 40 mg SQ every other week	Injection site reactions, infections	TB and hepatitis B tests must be performed prior to initiating since increased risk of TB and hepatitis B; possible to develop either intolerance or nonresponse over time
400 mg SQ wks 2, 4, then every 4 wks	Injection site reactions, infections	TB and hepatitis B tests must be performed prior to initiating since increased risk of TB and hepatitis B; possible to develop either intolerance or nonresponse over time

Name	Class	FDA IBD indication	Common uses	
Golimumab (Simponi)	Biologic agent (anti-TNF)	UC	Moderate to severe UC	
Vedolizumab (Entyvio)	Biologic agent (anti-alpha 4 beta 7 integrin)	Inflammatory CD, UC	Moderate to severe CD, UC	
Ustekinumab (Stelara)	Biologic agent (anti-IL12, 23)	Inflammatory CD, UC	Moderate to severe CD, UC	
Tofacitinib (Xeljancz)	Small molecule, nonselective JAK kinase inhibitor	Moderate to severe UC after failure of anti-TNF	Moderate to severe UC	
Ozanimod (Zeposia)	Small molecule, anti-S1P	Moderate to severe UC	Active UC	

Dosing	Common adverse events	Special considerations
200 mg SQ wk 0,100 mg wk 2, then 100 mg every 4 weeks	Injection site reactions, infection	TB and hepatitis B tests must be performed prior to initiating since increased risk of TB and hepatitis B; possible to develop either intolerance or nonresponse over time
300 mg IV wks 0, 2, 6, then every 8 wks	Infection but no signal for PML	Formal testing for TB and hepatitis B not necessary but often performed
Dose ranging via IV once, then 90 mg SQ every 8 wks	Injection site reactions, infection	TB testing must be performed prior to initiating since increased risk of TB; possible to develop either intolerance or nonresponse over time
5 mg or 10 mg twice a day	Shingles infection, blood clots	TB and hepatitis B tests must be performed prior to initiating since increased risk of TB and hepatitis B; ideally receive shingles vaccine SHINGRIX before starting
Gradual increase in dose over 1 wk starting with 0.23 mg	URI, headache, slowed heart rate	Screening for heart arrhythmia and eye conditions prior to starting

MEDICATIONS FOR SPECIFIC SYMPTOMS

It's not uncommon for individuals with IBD to take medications to treat specific symptoms associated with the disease as opposed to drugs designed to manage their condition. Diarrhea and pain are common symptoms of IBD so, not surprisingly, antidiarrheals and pain medications are frequently prescribed for people with ulcerative colitis and Crohn's disease.

Antidiarrheals

There are several different antidiarrheals available, some sold over the counter and others available by prescription. Loperamide (Imodium) comes in pill, capsule and liquid forms as well as in combination with anti-gas agents. Whether you buy loperamide over the counter or receive it by prescription, the strength is the same.

Loperamide acts in two ways to stop diarrhea: It slows the muscular activity of the gut, and it strengthens the tone of the anal sphincter. Generally, doses are in the range of 2 to 16 milligrams a day.

Diphenoxylate-atropine (Lomotil) is available by prescription only and works differently than loperamide. A combination of two drugs, diphenoxylate-atropine slows down contractions of the intestines. The recommended dose is two to eight tablets a day.

The best way to take loperamide or diphenoxylate-atropine is before meals, because meals stimulate movement of waste through the GI tract and evacuation. If you take the pills after you eat or have a loose stool, it's already too late. If you have chronic diarrhea or frequent loose stools, you need to take either medication before the diarrhea for it to be most effective. Because these two medications work in different ways, they're sometimes used in combination with each other or other antidiarrheals.

The antidiarrheal cholestyramine (Colestid, Welchol) binds bile. Extra bile can flow to the colon because of intestinal surgery or you've had your gallbladder removed. Bile is a direct irritant to the colon wall and causes watery diarrhea. Cholestyramine binds the extra bile to remove it, which results in firmer stools. It can be taken up to four times a day,

Tammy is 45 years old and has had three surgeries for her Crohn's disease. She's on 6-MP medications with good control of her inflammation, but because of her surgeries, she has chronic diarrhea. Tammy takes loperamide on a regular basis: two tablets each morning and evening, and sometimes one in the middle of the day. She's experimented over the years with how many pills she needs to take at a time and has figured out what works best for her.

depending on the amount of bile that's reaching the colon.

Tincture of opium alleviates diarrhea by slowing the muscular activity of the intestines. It's not used if you're prone to intestinal obstructions. The medication comes in drops that you add to water and drink several times daily. This medication causes drowsiness, and because it's a controlled substance, it requires a written prescription that must be renewed monthly. Also, if you take this medication and undergo a urine test, the test will come back positive for illegal drugs. Tincture of opium is probably third or fourth on the list of medications to try for diarrhea because of its side effects and because it's a regulated drug.

Codeine is a pain medication that also treats diarrhea. A side effect of its pain-killing actions is that it also slows down the motor contractions of the intestines. Codeine is less habit forming than other narcotics, but again, it's a third or fourth choice because, as a controlled substance, it will produce a positive drug test and can become addictive.

Teduglutide (GATTEX) is a hormone that helps grow small intestinal cells and is used in patients who are dependent on intravenous fluids and feedings to survive. This is a unique medication intended for individuals with only a limited amount of small intestine remaining following surgery to remove damaged intestine (short bowel syndrome). Teduglutide can help reduce the need for intravenous support and reduce the number of stools per day.

Pain medications

Active symptoms of IBD are often painful, so learning how to manage pain is important, and that often includes use of medication. The most important thing to remember is that pain medication is meant to be used for relatively short amounts of time. Long-term use may lead to side effects, and some medications can be addictive in nature.

Acetaminophen (Tylenol) is the preferred over-the-counter pain medication because it won't upset your stomach like other pain relievers can. Nonsteroidal anti-inflammatory drugs (NSAIDs) are the other common class of over-the-counter pain medicines. They include ibuprofen (Advil, Motrin) and naproxen sodium (Aleve). These drugs can cause inflammation and ulceration of the stomach and small and large intestines. For that reason, they should be avoided if possible.

Several studies suggest that regular use of NSAIDs can increase the risk of active disease (a flare) as much as 30%. NSAIDs work differently than anti-inflammatories used to treat ulcerative colitis and Crohn's disease. There are two major biochemical pathways that cause inflammation. NSAIDs help control pain by affecting the other inflammatory process — not the one associated with IBD medications. When absolutely needed, such as after a dental procedure, conservative use of NSAIDs, with food, for the shortest time possible is OK.

Tramadol (Ultram) is a nonnarcotic pain medication taken orally. Doctors generally prefer it to narcotics because it doesn't have as much addictive potential and is safer than NSAIDs. Ketorolac (Toradol) is a pain medication commonly given in hospital emergency departments for acute pain. Because ketorolac has been associated with kidney damage in people with IBD, doctors avoid using it.

Narcotics such as oxycodone, meperidine and morphine may be prescribed to treat severe pain from active disease or after surgery. Once the active inflammation causing the pain is under control, the drugs should be discontinued. It's very important to wean yourself off narcotics as soon as possible.

Many people with Crohn's disease experience pain even when there's no evidence of active disease. This may be due to overactive nerve stimulation affecting the bowel wall that has occurred from years of active disease. This type of pain should be treated with nonnarcotic pain medications and other nonmedicinal interventions, perhaps in conjunction with a pain specialist.

If you have ulcerative colitis, narcotics can slow the bowel enough to make a sick colon even worse. In the case of bad cramping, it might be better to take antianxiety medications to help you relax rather than drugs that slow the bowel.

If you're experiencing intense, sharp pain, this could be a more serious problem, such as an impending bowel perforation (similar to what happens with appendicitis), and you should seek immediate medical care.

Several states have approved medical marijuana (cannabis) to treat Crohn's disease as well as pain and nausea. The marijuana may come in liquid, edible or tobacco form. The studies involving marijuana as a treatment for Crohn's disease suggest that it's helpful for symptoms. It may decrease pain and improve appetite, but there's no proof it's associated with decreasing inflammation and healing of the lining of the intestines. A lot more research is needed before we fully understand its safety and effectiveness. If you use medical marijuana, let your medical team know.

FUTURE TREATMENTS

Researchers are continually learning more about the mechanisms of inflammation in IBD, which will eventually lead to the development of new drugs. There are currently several different treatment approaches under investigation, including technology that will allow bacteria to deliver healthy proteins directly to the intestinal wall. Treatments that haven't been studied in large trials, sometimes used as last-ditch efforts to control Crohn's disease and ulcerative colitis, are also awaiting exploration. In short, the work continues.

Upcoming therapies

Several new treatments are expected to be approved by the FDA in the near future — some possibly before publication of this book. They include the following therapies.

Upadacitinib and filgotinib

These drugs are known as Janus kinase (JAK) inhibitors. JAK inhibitors are made up of small molecule compounds that are broken down in the gastrointestinal (GI) tract after ingestion. Once broken down, the compounds block multiple messaging pathways to control inflammation. The JAK inhibitor tofacitinib is already approved for treatment of ulcerative colitis. Upadacitinib (Rinvoq) — approved for rheumatoid arthritis, psoriatic arthritis and atopic dermatitis — and filgotinib may have fewer side effects than tofacitinib because they're more targeted (but can be just as effective).

Risankizumab

This drug is marketed as Skyrizi and is FDA approved for the treatment of psoriasis and psoriatic arthritis. It's similar to the drug ustekinumab in that it inhibits an interleukin, but only IL-23 and not both IL-12 and IL-23. Again, the thought is that if a treatment is more targeted, it may be safer.

Mirikizumab

This medication is another anti-IL-23 blocker similar to risankizumab. It's being studied in clinical trials.

Stool-based products

Fecal microbial transplants (stool transplants, or FMT) are FDA approved for the treatment of recurrent *C. difficile* infections. They've been used in several studies to treat both adults and children with IBD. Results are mixed and seem to be dependent on the composition of donor stool, mode of administration and number of times given. Another fecal-based therapy under active investigation is SER-287, a spore-based capsule for mild ulcerative colitis.

Stem cells for fistulas

Stem cells are cells that have the potential to become any kind of cell in the body. These cells are embedded on either a plug or string and implanted into an abnormal connection or tunnel (fistula). There, the cells mature into connective tissue and close the fistula. Early use has shown promising results in the treatment of perianal fistulas from Crohn's disease.

Hyperbaric oxygen

Hyperbaric oxygen is used to treat skin wounds, such as severe burns. Among some people with IBD, the colon or a fistula can contain a large amount of inflammation. Researchers are studying whether sitting in a hyperbaric oxygen chamber can aid tissue healing and reduce inflammation.

CLINICAL TRIALS

Perhaps the medications that you've tried haven't worked or have stopped working. Or perhaps the medications worked but the side effects were too severe. Maybe you're stuck on steroids, and you can't seem to get off them. These are all reasons you might consider joining a clinical trial.

At any given time, there are multiple trials underway at different research centers across the country. In the past 10 years, clinical trials have produced medications that are more targeted and better at treating IBD, and more are in the pipeline. None of the therapies currently used to treat IBD would be available if it hadn't been for clinical trials.

Participating in a clinical trial offers several advantages:
- You're receiving cutting-edge therapy that isn't otherwise available.
- Associated medical care is free of charge to you, and you may even receive some money for your time and effort.
- You're helping advance the science and care of IBD.
- It may be an opportunity to prove to yourself that you've tried everything before undergoing surgery.

All clinical trials, regardless of their size or funding source, must be listed on the government's clinical trials website. This site and the Crohn's & Colitis Foundation website are excellent resources for learning about clinical trials taking place in your area (see page 183). In addition, all clinical trials are first approved by ethics review boards not affiliated with the investigators or the pharmaceutical companies.

STAYING ON YOUR MEDICATION

So, you're finally feeling better, and you may be wondering if you need to continue to take your medication now that your symptoms are gone. After all, it's been a while (thankfully) since you've had an IBD flare.

The answer is yes, you need to stay on your medications. It's very important to continue taking them. Here's a partial list of the reasons why:
- IBD is a chronic, incurable disease, just like diabetes. You wouldn't encourage your brother who has diabetes to stop taking his insulin just because he feels well.
- There may still be inflammation in your digestive tract, even if you feel well. This may get the better of you if you let it. Medications help slow down the inflammatory process and promote healing, which ultimately leads to fewer potential future complications.
- People with IBD who discontinue their medications — even for a short time — have earlier relapses than people who stay on them. This is particularly true if you've needed long courses of steroids in the past.
- Discontinuing your medications can lead to more aggressive flares, which may require steroid therapy, hospitalization or surgery.
- A long-term study performed at the University of Chicago followed patients for two years. It found a fivefold increased risk of a disease flare of ulcerative colitis if the patients took less than 80% of their prescribed medication (mesalamine). Those who stayed on

their medications were less likely to visit a doctor or undergo procedures and ultimately saved money.

- Two studies have shown that patients with Crohn's disease on long-term azathioprine therapy are at risk of a flare if they stop taking the drug, even when they've been well (flare-free) for more than five years.
- Several studies have shown that taking 5-ASA medications over the long term may decrease your risk of developing cancer. It's unclear whether this protection is due to controlling inflammation or is a separate effect altogether.
- Long-term clinical trials have demonstrated that remaining on biologics and small molecules (tofacitinib and ozanimod) lowers the risk of relapse.

What are some reasons to stop something that's working for you? Maybe your health care providers haven't done a good job of explaining what your medications do and why you need to continue their use. Maybe the financial drain is overwhelming you. Maybe you think you can get by on a little less, so you're self-testing lower doses. Perhaps having IBD is a burden you'd rather not have to deal with. Or you keep forgetting to take your medications. You may have other reasons that are unique and private.

To avoid falling into an unhealthy situation, seek support from your health care team regarding your medications and your disease. The more you understand, the better. Here are some ideas about how to get support:

- Ask questions! If you don't understand what a medication does or what you should expect from it, then you're less likely to take it.
- If you're having trouble paying for your medications, ask about generic formulations and drug assistance programs.
- Ask your provider if you can take your medicines twice or even once a day, rather than multiple times, so that you don't forget.
- Keep small supplies of pills in several places so that when it's time to take them, you have some available.
- Know what to do if you miss a dose: Do you take the medication as soon as you remember, double up the next dose, or just take the next dose as you normally would? What are the consequences if you miss too many doses?
- Be open and honest with your health care providers about everything you're taking or using. They may not always like your choices, but at least they can watch out for unwanted or unexpected side effects from and interactions with the other substances.

COMPLEMENTARY THERAPIES

Some people look for answers to their health problems beyond those offered by their doctors. It's natural to want to know if a different approach can help you. Or perhaps you'd like more control over your disease and how it's being treated. Those are some of the reasons that people turn to unconventional treatments, often referred to as complementary, alternative or integrative medicine.

Most individuals turn to unconventional therapies not because they're dissatisfied with conventional medication but because they're looking for other ways to improve their condition and maintain their health. Complementary approaches tried by people with IBD fall into several categories:

- Diet.
- Exercise.
- Mind-body health: meditation, prayer, relaxation techniques, biofeedback.
- Physical manipulation: acupuncture, acupressure, chiropractic, massage.
- Oral therapy: vitamins, herbals, probiotics, homeopathy.

Doctors' primary concern regarding complementary approaches relates to your safety. They want their patients with IBD who use unconventional approaches to be informed about the therapy, its safety and how it works. Similar to any medication, the dosage, duration of use and potential interactions are all critical factors to be aware of. There generally aren't a lot of large, scientific studies involving complementary approaches. Unfortunately, many therapies rely primarily on anecdotal reports.

It's important to inform your health care providers if you're using an alternative approach, especially if you're taking anything orally. It's entirely possible that the agent you're ingesting is safe by itself, but when combined with other medications, it may not be. Also, two therapies individually may be fine, but put them together, and now it's not so fine. Consider peanut butter and tuna fish — separately they make fine sandwiches, but put them together and suddenly it isn't such a fine sandwich.

People often don't want to share information about the complementary therapies they're using because they worry their doctors may discount the benefits or be disappointed. The job of health care providers, as medical professionals, is to "do no harm." They don't want to prescribe or recommend drugs that might harm you because they're unaware of other things you're taking. Therefore, it's very important that you keep your health care provider aware of everything you use regarding your health.

Thoughts on certain therapies

This is what we know about some therapies used to manage IBD.

Aloe

Aloe is a popular homeopathic remedy believed by some to heal colitis. Unfortunately, the cells that line your colon aren't like those that line your skin, and there's no evidence it works for colitis. There are many forms of aloe, and some can be harmful to cells in the colon. Other extracts are being tested for their healing properties, but the research is still being done in rats and isn't ready for tests in humans. Because you can't tell which extract(s) may be in an aloe formulation, use it only on your skin and not for colitis.

Ginger

Ginger can soothe nausea, a common IBD symptom. Nausea may be due to a

THERAPIES NOT PROVEN TO WORK FOR IBD

Alternative medical systems

Ayurveda

Homeopathy

Naturopathy

Traditional Chinese medicine

Diet

FODMAP diet

Low-carbohydrate diet

Mediterranean diet

Paleo diet

Rice water diet

Specific carbohydrate diet

Oral therapies

Herbal supplements
- Aloe vera
- Bach Flower Remedies
- Boswellia serrata
- Calendula
- Cat's claw
- Chamomile
- Curcumin
- Ginseng
- Green tea
- Slippery elm
- Soy-derived isoflavones

Vitamin supplements

Mind-body interventions

Distant healing (sending compassionate thoughts via telepathic means)

Meditation

Prayer

Relaxation techniques

Physical therapy/exercise

Acupressure

Acupuncture

Aerobic exercise

Chiropractic/osteopathy

Feldenkrais

Hypnosis

Reiki therapy

Therapeutic touch

Probiotics/prebiotics

Align

Homeostatic soil organisms/primal defense

Nissle 1917

Probiotica

Saccharomyces boulardii

VSL#3

medication side effect or the disease itself. Drinking ginger ale can soothe nausea. Chewing on a piece of fresh ginger, chewing ginger gum or drinking ginger tea are all ways to relieve nausea. They're cheaper and safer than most of the drugs that treat nausea. Ginger is even safe to use during pregnancy and to give to small children.

Fish oil

Fish oil (omega-3 fatty acids) has been shown in a few studies to be helpful in treating mild to moderate Crohn's disease and ulcerative colitis. In those studies, 2 grams were needed to treat active disease, which is much stronger than what's sold in the United States. You'd need to eat about 12 pounds of fish a week to get that much omega-3. In addition, larger trials have failed to show any benefit from taking omega-3 to prevent flares. We don't recommend fish oil to treat IBD.

Curcumin

Curcumin, the ingredient in the spice turmeric, has anti-inflammatory properties. In small trials, it's been found to help maintain remission from flares, but so far it hasn't been shown to control disease in people with active symptoms.

The table on page 89 lists several complementary therapies. It's only a partial list, because the number of therapies people have experimented with to manage their IBD is too large to include.

With many of the therapies listed, there may not be enough reliable information to indicate whether they're helpful. So, the question is: Why spend money on something when there's no data indicating it works? If the attraction of these remedies is that they're "natural," a term often associated with complementary and alternative medicine, remember that you wouldn't sit in a patch of poison ivy or play with jellyfish even though those are 100% natural. Natural doesn't mean safe.

Probiotics

Probiotic therapy has been studied as a treatment for IBD. Probiotics are the "good" bacteria that normally live in your gastrointestinal (GI) tract. In addition to promoting colon health, they assist with the last stages of digestion. A popular theory is that with IBD, the natural balance of good bacteria is disrupted and needs to be replenished. The idea is that eating foods or taking supplements that contain so-called good bacteria can improve digestive health by replacing "bad" bacteria.

There are millions of strains of bacteria in the human colon, and it's hard to know which ones are the most important. However, we know that some, such as the *acidophilus*, *lactobacillus* and *bifidobacterium* species, have anti-inflammatory properties. Literally hundreds of probiotic formulas are available, some with just one strain and others with multiple strains. Just as one perfume or cologne may not be right for everyone, there isn't a one-size-fits-all solution for probiotics.

You may have to try several formulations before you find one that seems to help. Probiotics sold as supplements in health food stores contain 10^9-10^{10} (1-10 billion) organisms per dose. While seemingly a large amount, one gram of stool contains 1×10^{12} (one trillion) bacteria.

Don't be afraid to try probiotics. Here are some points to keep in mind:

- While probiotics can help, they shouldn't be your sole therapy for IBD.
- For many people, probiotics improve the symptoms of bloating, gas and some of the cramping, and they may help with irregularity.
- A probiotic can give you GI symptoms, depending on how it reacts with your digestive system. Do your homework about which one to use, and be clear about your goals.
- Because probiotics are bacteria, they need to be ingested live or else they're useless. They're protected from stomach acid by the outer coating of the capsule they come in or because of their natural defenses. Make sure the brand you buy has an expiration date and has been through some sort of quality control, as evidenced by a batch number on the box.
- Products can range from a generic single species per capsule to combination capsules. There are products marketed by pharmaceutical companies that do have to abide by the rigors of quality control. Some examples include Align, Flora-Stor, Flora-Q and VSL#3.
- You need to take probiotics on a regular basis, or their effects wear off. If you can't use them consistently, don't use them at all.

- If you're having gastrointestinal symptoms and try a probiotic and your symptoms persist, stop the probiotic and mention this to your health care provider.
- Probiotics don't cure or prevent disease. If you feel well, using them won't make you feel any better.

Prebiotics

Think of prebiotics as food for the good bacteria (probiotics) that reside in your gut. Prebiotics are the natural food components that help probiotics flourish. They're in essence the fertilizer that stimulates the growth of healthy bacteria. Prebiotics are found in a variety of foods, including asparagus, yams, banana, onions, garlic, legumes and whole-wheat products.

Research suggests prebiotics can help prevent and manage infectious and antibiotic-resistant diarrhea and reduce symptoms associated with some gastrointestinal diseases. Prebiotics are now being looked at as potential alternatives to some traditional IBD therapies. However, as with any medicine, the particular species and dose are critical, and more research is needed.

7

IBD affects more than your gut

When your gastrointestinal (GI) tract isn't healthy, which is the case with IBD, almost every part of your body can be affected. This chapter looks at how your disease may present itself in other parts of your body.

EYES

Two eye conditions in particular are associated with IBD: uveitis and iritis. Fortunately, they're relatively uncommon, occurring in less than 5% of people with the disease.

Uveitis is inflammation of the middle layer of the eye (uvea). The uvea consists of three structures: the iris, the ciliary body and the choroid. Iritis is inflammation of just one part of the uvea, the iris.

The iris regulates the amount of light entering the eye by changing the size of the pupil according to available light.

Both conditions can cause pain, a red appearance and blurred vision. Usually, only one eye is affected. It's typical for either uveitis or iritis to occur when you're experiencing active inflammation in your gut. Only an ophthalmologist, not an optometrist, can diagnose uveitis or iritis. These are serious conditions that need to be treated right away with eye drops that control the inflammation.

Other eye conditions can develop as side effects of some IBD medications. The most common are cataracts, caused by prolonged steroid use, and pink eye (conjunctivitis), which is more frequent when taking immunosuppressants because the drugs interfere with your ability to fight common infections.

LIVER

There are two liver diseases that may occur in people with IBD. One is known as primary sclerosing cholangitis. The other is autoimmune hepatitis.

Primary sclerosing cholangitis

In this condition, the walls of the liver's bile ducts become inflamed (cholangitis). The condition eventually leads to narrowing of and damage to the bile ducts. Bile ducts are the passageways that carry bile from the liver. Chronic inflammation in the ducts can eventually lead to severe scarring of the liver, known as cirrhosis. Complications of cirrhosis include liver failure and liver cancer.

Primary sclerosing cholangitis is usually discovered when blood tests suggest an abnormality in liver enzymes. Otherwise, there are few, if any, symptoms until the disease has progressed. A diagnosis is generally made by way of a test called magnetic resonance cholangiopancreatography (MRCP), in which images are taken of the liver and bile ducts.

Another diagnostic tool is a procedure called endoscopic retrograde cholangiopancreatography (ERCP). In this procedure dye is injected into the bile ducts and images are taken of the ducts. In some situations, a liver biopsy may be performed.

The severity of primary sclerosing cholangitis doesn't parallel IBD activity. Even when IBD is under control, the bile ducts inside and outside the liver can be actively inflamed, or vice versa. About 5% of people with IBD develop primary sclerosing cholangitis. However, sometimes primary sclerosing cholangitis is found first. It turns out that about 80% to 90% of individuals with primary sclerosing cholangitis have some sort of underlying IBD.

To date, we don't have an effective treatment for primary sclerosing cholangitis or a way to prevent it or predict who might get it. Some doctors use a bile salt called ursodiol to help control the inflammation. Although ursodiol can improve liver enzyme elevations and liver inflammation and damage in some people, it's uncertain if the medication can stop the progression of primary sclerosing cholangitis, and high doses may be dangerous.

The nature of the disease is variable: Some people never experience any symptoms but clearly have abnormalities on imaging studies or blood tests. Others experience progressive primary sclerosing cholangitis that causes such severe damage that they may need a liver transplant.

Autoimmune hepatitis

With autoimmune hepatitis, your immune system begins to attack your liver, causing inflammation and damage. It's similar to what happens in your GI tract when your IBD is active. Symptoms of autoimmune hepatitis range from none at all to severe liver damage requiring a liver transplant. Autoimmune hepatitis is treated with medications that control inflammation, typically a combination of steroids and azathioprine.

Other liver-related issues

Medications taken to treat IBD — including azathioprine, 6-MP, methotrexate and, in rare instances, sulfasalazine or some biologics — can harm the liver. If you have a hepatitis B infection, you shouldn't receive certain biologic therapies until the hepatitis is treated, because the medication can make the infection worse. Taking too much acetaminophen (Tylenol), which is commonly used to control pain from Crohn's disease, can damage the liver. You shouldn't combine acetaminophen with alcohol.

Gallstones that form in the gallbladder, where bile from the liver is stored, are more common in people with Crohn's disease, as well as in individuals who need prolonged intravenous feeding (total parenteral nutrition, or TPN). Over the long term, TPN can also cause fat to be deposited in the liver, producing liver damage.

TPN may serve as therapy for Crohn's disease, particularly in people who have a large amount of inflammation in the small intestine or large fistulas involving the bowel and skin. It provides calories and nutrition to individuals with Crohn's disease who can't get adequate calories from their daily diets.

KIDNEYS

People with Crohn's disease are more susceptible to developing kidney stones. This is because Crohn's affects the body's ability to get rid of excess oxalate, a nutrient found in many foods. When diarrhea or inflammation is present, the body loses calcium, and calcium is what binds oxalate in the intestines. With inadequate calcium, oxalate is free to be absorbed back into the bloodstream.

From the bloodstream, oxalate is deposited in the kidneys because it has nowhere else to go. As the oxalate builds up, it forms stones. These stones may travel out of the kidney with urine, damaging the urinary tract and causing bleeding and pain. You may know someone who's passed a kidney stone. The pain it causes is compared to childbirth. It comes on suddenly and is felt on one side of the back.

Treatment of kidney stones includes oral and intravenous fluid to flush the stone through the system. Sometimes, a urologist threads a small, flexible scope (cystoscope) up into the bladder and extracts a stone that's stuck. Some people may have kidney stones broken up with ultrasound sonic waves. Taking extra calcium supplements helps prevent oxalate from being reabsorbed, and it's one of the simplest and best treatments.

Some medications used to treat IBD can potentially affect the kidneys. Specifically, 5-ASA medications can produce a type of kidney damage called idiosyncratic, which means there's no rhyme or reason for the damage; it can occur at any time and at any dose. Even though this is relatively rare, if you use 5-ASA therapy, your doctor will monitor your kidney function with blood tests — initially every two to 12 weeks, and then usually every six to 12 months. In rare cases, Crohn's disease and ulcerative colitis may trigger certain autoimmune kidney diseases.

BONES

The rate of osteoporosis is higher among individuals with IBD compared to the general population. Osteoporosis is a bone disease that causes bones to become abnormally thin and brittle. If you have osteoporosis, you're at increased risk of fracturing bones in your wrist, ribs, spine and hips. These breaks can occur with even a minor injury.

Osteopenia is an early stage of bone thinning in which your bones are weaker than normal, but not so much that they break as easily as they do with osteoporosis.

More than 10 million Americans have osteoporosis, resulting in 1.5 million fractures per year. Another 43 million Americans have osteopenia. Most people with osteoporosis and osteopenia are women, but the disorders do affect men. Studies show that people with IBD, especially those with Crohn's disease, are at increased risk of osteopenia and eventually osteoporosis. Some estimates suggest that osteoporosis occurs in 1 in 7 people with Crohn's disease and that

nearly half of all those with Crohn's have osteopenia.

The most important risk factors for osteoporosis in the general population — older age, being female and having a low body mass index — are still the most important predictors of osteoporosis among individuals with IBD. Here are some additional reasons why osteoporosis is more common among individuals with IBD.

- Corticosteroids, such as prednisone, have powerful effects on bone metabolism. In fact, decreased bone density and increased fracture risk may occur within a few months of starting steroids. Even low-dose prednisone — 5 milligrams daily — is associated with fracture risk.
- Immunomodulators, such as cyclosporine and methotrexate, may reduce bone density slightly.
- IBD itself, especially Crohn's disease, may be a risk factor. Low bone densities have been noted in newly diagnosed patients, even before being treated with corticosteroids. It's possible that higher protein levels associated with inflammation have negative effects on bone formation and speed bone loss.
- When Crohn's disease involves the small intestine or there's been removal (resection) of the small intestine, you may be less able to absorb calcium and vitamin D, which are essential for strong bones.
- Many people with IBD have a low body mass index. This is an independent risk factor for osteoporosis.
- Cigarette smoking is a risk factor for osteoporosis, and many people with

Crohn's disease have a history of smoking or currently smoke.

People with IBD most at risk of fracture are postmenopausal women, those with low body mass index and those receiving steroids. Other risk factors include a history of heavy smoking, steroid treatment for at least three months at a time and prior fractures.

To monitor your risk, talk to your health care provider about a dual-energy X-ray absorptiometry (DEXA) scan to determine bone density. The results of a DEXA scan are usually given as a T-score. The T-score indicates how much different your bone density is from the general population's. Osteopenia is diagnosed when the T-score falls between -1.0 and -2.5, and osteoporosis is diagnosed when the T-score is below -2.5.

Preventing bone loss and bone fractures is an important goal for managing your IBD. To manage IBD-associated osteoporosis and reduce your risk of fractures, discuss these steps with your health care provider:
- Make healthy lifestyle changes, including exercising daily and stopping smoking.
- Get at least 1,200 milligrams of calcium daily. This can be a combination of dairy products and calcium carbonate or calcium citrate supplements.
- Take 400 to 800 international units (IUs) of vitamin D daily. You might need more if tests indicate you're low on vitamin D.
- If you take steroids, talk with your doctor about options for getting off of them and using medications such as azathioprine, 6-MP, methotrexate, small molecules and biologics.
- If you're postmenopausal, discuss hormone replacement therapy with your provider. Selective estrogen receptor modulators, such as raloxifene (Evista), may increase bone density and reduce fracture risk. However, this must be balanced with the increased risk of breast cancer associated with hormone replacement therapy.
- Consider taking bisphosphonates. Oral bisphosphonates — alendronate (Fosamax) and risedronate (Actonel), for example — may be administered either on a daily or weekly basis. Both medications have been shown to increase back and neck bone density and reduce back and hip fractures for both postmenopausal and glucocorticoid-induced osteoporosis. In addition, risedronate prevents bone loss in individuals receiving corticosteroids. However, some GI side effects, including inflammation of the esophagus, can occasionally occur with either medication.
- Discuss other preparations, such as pamidronate (Aredia) or zoledronic acid (Zometa) if you can't tolerate oral bisphosphonates. Pamidronate is given intravenously every three to six months. Zoledronic acid is given once a year.
- If you're more than five years postmenopausal, consider nasal salmon calcitonin spray (Miacalcin), which can effectively improve bone density and reduce fractures in the lower back. Calcitonin is a hormone important for bone health, and salmon extracts are an easy source.

Another condition that can affect your bones is osteomalacia. This condition is different from osteoporosis and osteopenia in that it results from nutritional deficiencies rather than bone thinning due to calcium loss. Osteomalacia can be reversed if the reason behind it is identified and corrected.

JOINTS

When your gut is sick, it can make your joints hurt too. Aching or pain in the joints associated with IBD is called arthralgia. This is different from arthritis, which is inflammation in a joint that damages the joint over time. There's no damage to the joints with IBD-associated arthralgia. The pain can occur in large or smaller joints of the body — hands, knees and ankles — and usually the pain parallels the IBD activity in the gut. The pain can move from one joint to another, so you may have painful ankles that over time feel better, but then you experience pain in a hip during another flare.

Arthralgia can also occur during steroid withdrawal, but this pain lasts only a few days as the dose is decreased. Painful joints may also result from azathioprine use. If you stop the medication, the pain will go away. Arthralgia is treated by managing active gut symptoms. Certain IBD medications may help reduce joint pain, including sulfasalazine, methotrexate, tofacitinib and the anti-TNF agents (see Chapter 6).

There are two arthritic conditions in which there's destruction of the joint and bone — ankylosing spondylitis and sacroiliitis. These large joint conditions can cause hip and back pain. Unlike arthralgia, the conditions follow their own course and don't parallel inflammation in the gut. Ankylosing spondylitis and sacroiliitis are treated with medications similar to those used for rheumatoid arthritis.

Steroid use can also damage joints and cause pain. Steroids may lead to a condition called avascular necrosis (AVN), in which blood vessels that feed the center of the bone die, creating joint pain and eventually destroying the joint. The best way to prevent this condition is to wean yourself from steroids as soon as possible.

HAIR, TEETH AND NAILS

Your hair and nails are the last parts of your body to receive nutrition. So, if you're sick, they can become unhealthy rather quickly. Hair thinning or hair loss can occur because of an iron deficiency, a delayed reaction to a flare even months after the flare is under control, and ongoing active disease. IBD medications associated with hair loss include steroids, high doses of 5-ASAs, azathioprine, methotrexate and biologics.

Healthy nails depend on good nutrition. Vitamin and mineral deficiencies as well as active disease can cause delayed nail growth, brittle or easily broken nails and nail discoloration.

Diseases of the gums and teeth and poor oral health may also result from Crohn's disease. This is generally due to ongoing inflammation in the gums, poor nutrition and steroid use. Diseases of the gums and teeth may also be a side effect of smoking. Chronic vomiting can cause dental erosion from exposure to excessive amounts of stomach acid.

SKIN

Some medications used to treat Crohn's disease and ulcerative colitis can affect the skin. Steroids can result in thinning of the skin, which causes easy bruising and stretch marks (striae). Steroids may also cause or worsen acne.

Rarely, the medication methotrexate is associated with development of skin nodules. If you notice skin changes while on methotrexate, mention it to your health care provider. The nodules will eventually go away if you stop taking methotrexate, but your provider needs to make this adjustment; you may be prescribed a new medication.

Two skin rashes — known as erythema nodosum and pyoderma gangrenosum — are associated with Crohn's disease and ulcerative colitis.

Erythema nodosum

This is a painful condition in which red nodules appear on the shins and ankles. About 15% of people with IBD develop this condition, and it occurs with several other autoimmune conditions as well. Erythema nodosum may develop before

other signs and symptoms of IBD become apparent. It parallels the activity of the GI tract: Treat the inflammation in the gut, and the skin gets better.

Erythema nodosum starts off looking like a bruise but then gets redder and more painful, sometimes so painful that it's hard to walk. This is such a well-known skin condition that, generally, your doctor won't need to take a biopsy to make a diagnosis. The condition can sometimes be confused with Sweet's disease, which is another skin condition characterized by itchy red bumps, but mostly on the upper body. Sweet's disease is an autoimmune condition. It's rare in people with IBD, but it also tends to parallel the gut activity.

Pyoderma gangrenosum

This skin condition occurs in about 5% of individuals with IBD. It usually affects the legs but can also occur on the arm or around a skin opening (stoma). It's not fully understood why this skin condition happens more often among people with IBD.

Pyoderma gangrenosum starts off as a little bump that can look like a bug bite. It gets bigger and bigger, particularly if you pick at it: The more you pick, the bigger the bump gets. Over time, the bump turns into an ulcer-like crater, which is painful. Any manipulation of the area, such as taking a biopsy, makes it worse.

This condition runs its own course and doesn't parallel inflammation in the gut.

Conditions that accompany inflammation of the GI tract	Conditions that don't accompany inflammation of the GI tract
Arthralgias	Ankylosing spondylitis
Erythema nodosum	Sacroiliitis
Iritis	Autoimmune hepatitis
Uveitis	Primary sclerosing cholangitis
Sweet's disease	Pyoderma gangrenosum

Without treatment, it will continue to get worse, resulting in multiple ulcers. If you catch pyoderma gangrenosum while the bump is small, sometimes it can be cleared up with a prescription skin cream (tacrolimus, Protopic). Otherwise, it is controlled with medications to treat the gut, such as steroids, azathioprine, and anti-TNF agents. The ulcers usually leave a scar after they've healed.

The IBD-cancer connection

Colon cancer, also known as colorectal cancer, occurs in about 33 in 100,000 people in the United States. Having IBD increases your risk of colorectal cancer twofold, to about 60 in 100,000. Colorectal cancer is a relatively rare complication of IBD, but because there's a connection it's important to be extra vigilant and monitor for it. Colorectal cancer can be prevented, and self-management is the key.

Most cases of colorectal cancer can be traced to a colon polyp, an inward bulge of the colon lining that becomes cancerous. Colorectal cancer in IBD arises from precancerous dysplasia. Unlike the easier-to-identify polyps in people who don't have Crohn's disease or ulcerative colitis, dysplasia associated with IBD may occur in the flat lining of the colon.

IBD dysplasia is more difficult to see during a colonoscopy. Therefore, in addition to taking random biopsies throughout the colon to identify dysplasia, your gastroenterologist may use a technique called chromoendoscopy, in which a dye is sprayed throughout the colon during a colonoscopy. Some medical providers feel that chromoendoscopy is a more efficient way of identifying precancerous changes associated with IBD.

CANCER RISK

Your specific risk for colorectal cancer depends on how much damage has occurred in the colon and how long the damage has been present. Most studies have looked at colorectal cancer risk in individuals with ulcerative colitis, but people with Crohn's disease involving the colon (Crohn's colitis) are also at increased risk.

Risk of colorectal cancer increases with IBD duration. In older studies, the risk was estimated at approximately 2% after 10 years of disease, 8% after 20 years and as high as 20% by 30 years of disease. The good news is that more recent studies have demonstrated a lower risk of developing colorectal cancer, which is attributed to more aggressive treatment of IBD.

Risk factors for dysplasia and colorectal cancer include some things that you have no control over. They include how long you've had IBD, how severe or extensive your disease is and a family history of colorectal cancer, independent of your disease. The younger you are at diagnosis also seems to increase your risk.

Another risk factor that's beyond your control is having primary sclerosing cholangitis. It's unclear why having primary sclerosing cholangitis makes a person more susceptible to colon cancer, because other liver diseases don't increase the risk.

However, there is one important risk factor that you do have control over — the degree of inflammation within the intestines, which can be controlled by aggressive medical care and self-management. Properly managing your IBD appears to offer promise for lowering your risk of developing colorectal cancer.

PREVENTING COLORECTAL CANCER

Most colorectal cancer associated with IBD can be prevented if both you and your health care team understand your individual risk and follow surveillance guidelines. In addition to the risk factors previously mentioned, your age weighs heavily in your overall risk, given that colorectal cancer increases with advancing age.

Guidelines from many health organizations, including the American College of Gastroenterology, American Gastroenterological Association and the American Society for Gastrointestinal Endoscopy, recommend that you undergo a surveillance colonoscopy with random biopsies or chromoendoscopy eight to 10 years after being diagnosed with IBD and that you repeat the procedure every one to three years, depending on the findings.

If you have primary sclerosing cholangitis, however, surveillance colonoscopy with random biopsies or chromoendoscopy should begin at the time of diagnosis and be repeated annually. For unknown reasons, polyps and cancer develop faster in people with primary sclerosing cholangitis than in people with IBD who don't have that condition.

Undergoing so many colonoscopies may seem like a lot of effort, unpleasant prep, and expense, but they can save your life. If doctors find precancerous dysplasia, they can get rid of it. If colorectal cancer is identified at an earlier stage, the chance of a cure is greatly increased. When colorectal cancer isn't found early, it can become invasive and much more difficult to cure.

Studies show that in people who regularly undergo surveillance colonoscopy, colorectal cancer is more likely to be discovered early, when it's still dysplasia. Other ways to reduce your cancer risk are by managing your disease and avoiding flares.

DEALING WITH DYSPLASIA

Dysplasia is a change in the structure of the cells lining the intestine that occurs prior to the development of cancer. Low-grade dysplasia typically develops first. It can revert to normal tissue, stay constant or progress to high-grade dysplasia. Doctors don't understand all the factors that determine which direction low-grade dysplasia will take, but having continued active inflammation is a known risk factor for dysplasia and cancer.

Dysplasia is further classified by how many places it's found within the colon. If it's located only in one location, it's called unifocal. If it's in multiple places, it's called multifocal. Management of multifocal dysplasia is much more aggressive than that of unifocal dysplasia because the chances of the dysplasia progressing to cancer are much higher when the condition is in multiple places.

If your colonoscopy reveals dysplasia, have the biopsies read by a second pathologist — if possible, someone who's an expert in the field. The gastroenterolo-

Eloise had a long history of Crohn's disease of the colon and underwent regular colonoscopies. When she was 55, doctors found a small bump on the right side of her rectum that easily could have been missed without good preparation and a thorough procedure. The bump was biopsied and found to be very early cancer. Because it was found at such an early stage, and because the traditional treatment approach meant Eloise would lose her colon and need a permanent colostomy bag, she opted for more specialized tissue removal plus increased surveillance with more frequent colonoscopies. This isn't an option for everyone, but, fortunately, it was easy to completely remove Eloise's tumor without surgery. Three years later, another area of cancer was found, and this time there was no doubt that Eloise's colon had to be removed. She was grateful for the three years in which she was able to postpone the operation, and even more grateful that the second cancer was found early as well.

gist who took your biopsies can send your slides for the consultation without your having to travel. If a second pathologist agrees that you have dysplasia, you might talk with your doctor about a referral to an IBD specialty center if you aren't already visiting such a center.

It's important to discuss your options with professionals who treat IBD complications, including colorectal cancer, every day. The decision about the next steps to take is highly individualized and is based on your health history, family history of polyps and cancer, other medical conditions you may have and your personal preferences. You'll need to decide whether to undergo frequent follow-up colonoscopies or have surgery.

If the dysplasia is found in a polyp, removing the polyp and undergoing regular follow-up colonoscopies — approximately every six to 12 months, initially — may be enough to keep you safe. Again, the decision about how to manage and treat dysplasia is dependent on a lot of factors, and a second opinion is always worthwhile in this situation. This is especially true if your colitis is under control and your doctor is recommending surgery. During these discussions, however, don't lose sight of the fact that colorectal cancer is curable in its earliest stages.

MEDICATIONS TO PREVENT COLORECTAL CANCER

A number of medications may help prevent development of dysplasia and colorectal cancer in people with long-standing colitis. Taking 1 milligram of folic acid a day as a supplement has been shown to decrease the risk of dysplasia in ulcerative colitis. Adequate folic acid intake isn't difficult to achieve in the United States because it's a common additive in food and is found in almost all multivitamins.

The mainstay of treatment for mild ulcerative colitis, 5-ASA medications play a key role in preventing dysplasia and colorectal cancer. In several studies, using 5-ASA at doses of 1.2 grams per day or greater reduced the risk of cancer by 72% to 80%. Although more research is needed, keep in mind that in addition to reversing inflammation in ulcerative colitis and maintaining remission of inflammation, 5-ASAs may protect against colorectal cancer.

Additional data suggest that other medications used to treat IBD, including 6-MP and biologics, may lower your risk of developing colorectal cancer if they can heal the lining of your colon.

OTHER TYPES OF CANCER

In addition to colorectal cancer, there is evidence that some medications used to treat IBD may increase your risk of other cancers.

Lymphoma

Lymphoma is cancer of the T and B white blood cells (lymphocytes) that make up the lymph nodes. The two major kinds of lymphoma — Hodgkin's lymphoma and non-Hodgkin's lymphoma — are diagnosed according to what these cells look like under the microscope and their genetic makeup.

Among Americans, the risk of developing lymphoma is age dependent. The rate is 2 to 3 per 100,000 people between ages 19 and 25 and rises to 39 to 54 per 100,000 individuals after age 60.

Many potential risk factors for lymphoma have been noted, including *Helicobacter pylori* infection, exposure to certain pesticides, and certain autoimmune diseases such as rheumatoid arthritis, Sjogren's syndrome, and even IBD itself. Taking the medications 6-MP and azathioprine increase the risk of developing lymphoma. In a study from France, patients who took medications that suppress the immune system — such as azathioprine and 6-MP and biologic agents used to treat IBD — were more likely to develop lymphoma over time. The increased risk was between 2 and 4 times higher than the general population.

Because the risk of lymphoma increases steadily with age, it's important to consider this connection as you get older. Most doctors believe that the benefits derived from controlling active IBD symptoms with immunosuppressive medications far outweigh the risk of developing lymphoma. Therefore, they continue to use the medications routinely for IBD and other autoimmune conditions.

Hepatosplenic T-cell lymphoma

Hepatosplenic T-cell lymphoma is seen in younger people, predominantly men, and is specifically associated with use of immunosuppressant drugs. Historically, this cancer was associated with azathioprine use, but recently it's been identified in a few patients taking both anti-TNFs and azathioprine. Hepatosplenic T-cell

Ryan had long-standing Crohn's disease of the small intestine. A routine appointment found that he had lost a few pounds. Ryan said that he hadn't noticed the weight loss but indicated that he was feeling a bit more tired, which he attributed to his job. At his next visit six months later, Ryan had lost more weight and said that he'd been sweating at night, which was new. An X-ray showed a new narrowing in his small intestine. He had surgery, which revealed that the narrowing was from lymphoma, rather than scar tissue associated with his disease. Ryan also had a few lymph nodes that tested positive for cancer. After a regimen of chemotherapy, he felt great and had more energy, and his weight returned to normal.

lymphoma is particularly aggressive, and unlike most other lymphomas it affects T cells rather than B cells. As a result, this disease doesn't respond well to chemotherapy medication and can be fatal.

Before doctors began prescribing anti-TNF drugs for children, hepatosplenic T-cell lymphoma was only seen in people taking azathioprine. But as use of the anti-TNF medications in children grew, so did the incidence of this lymphoma. Because this form of lymphoma is most often seen in people younger than age 20, there are now special warnings against use of anti-TNFs in younger patients, and many doctors have ceased using combinations of anti-TNFs and azathioprine or 6-MP to treat children with IBD.

Symptoms of lymphoma can be very nonspecific, and sometimes the cancer is discovered only because a CT scan shows a person's lymph nodes are enlarged. Symptoms can include anemia, fatigue, unexplained weight loss, night sweats and fever. Because a lot of other conditions can cause these symptoms, a complete physical examination is necessary, including feeling for any enlarged lymph glands in the neck area, armpits and groin. Individuals with IBD and lymphoma respond to chemotherapy in ways that are similar to how the rest of the population responds. After treatment, the lymphoma usually goes into remission.

Cholangiocarcinoma

Cholangiocarcinoma is cancer of the bile ducts. It's rare and usually associated with conditions that cause inflammation and scarring of the bile duct system, such as primary sclerosing cholangitis (see also Chapter 7). Therefore, if you have IBD and primary sclerosing cholangitis, you need to be monitored on a regular basis with blood tests that screen for changes in your liver enzymes, particularly an enzyme called alkaline phosphatase.

Usually there are no symptoms before the diagnosis is made. When a tumor affects the flow of bile, the typical result is yellowing of the skin and eyes (jaundice). Bile that can't flow properly can deposit in the skin and cause diffuse itching. Unexplained weight loss and vague abdominal pain may also occur.

Cholangiocarcinoma is diagnosed with imaging and a sampling of cells from the bile duct system. The cells usually are collected during a procedure called endoscopic retrograde cholangiopancreatography (ERCP), which combines uses of a thin, flexible tube (endoscope) and X-ray.

Cholangiocarcinoma is difficult to treat because it usually isn't found until it's advanced. If the cancer hasn't spread outside the liver, liver transplantation may be a treatment option.

Rare tumors

It's possible to develop cancer inside a fistula, but it's rare. If cancer occurs in a fistula in the perianal region, it may not be visible until it produces symptoms. If you've had a fistula for more than 10 to 15 years that hasn't healed, it's important to have it monitored for any change in its size or appearance.

Another rare cancer associated with Crohn's disease is cancer of the small intestine. Long-standing inflammation and scarring can produce abnormal cells that reproduce and develop into cancer similar to colorectal cancer. If you have Crohn's disease of the small intestine, it's important to undergo periodic monitoring with X-rays to look for changes that could signal cancer of the small intestine. Changes that may indicate cancer include irregular narrowing (stricture) or thickening of the intestinal wall.

There's no standard protocol for how often these tests should be done, because exposure to radiation without any symptoms is itself a risk. The increasing availability and use of MRI technology may help reduce this risk.

When you need surgery

Surgery is an important therapeutic tool in the management of IBD. In fact, in several situations, it has advantages over medications, so you shouldn't necessarily consider it to be a last resort. Sometimes, someone is so sick that it is best to perform surgery before other complications set in, such as a perforation or an infection. The job of doctors is to make patients better, and sometimes that's accomplished with surgery.

Take a few steps back here and look at the big picture by asking yourself a couple of questions. Have you worked your way through all your medication options without success? Is continuing your medication leading to more complications without the promise of improving your health? These are situations that you want to discuss with your doctor.

Let's say you have ulcerative colitis that hasn't gotten better despite trying many different medications or that only responds to high doses of steroids. You need to consider what you're achieving by walking around with a sick colon. It's also important to understand that a colon isn't an essential organ. Essential organs are the ones you can't live without — brain, heart, lungs, kidneys and liver.

Nobody wants to lose all or part of an organ, but when the organ is sick and you have little or no control over its function, daily living can become difficult. After having a sick colon removed, many of our patients say that they wish they hadn't waited so long to have surgery. They never realized how much their life was being compromised by carrying around such a burden. Once the colon has been removed, ulcerative colitis is essentially cured because with this disease, only the colon is involved.

For Crohn's disease, the story is different. One of the reasons that doctors may hesitate to recommend surgery for Crohn's disease is because the disease is likely to come back after surgery. It typically recurs at the place where the diseased bowel was removed and where the two healthy ends were reconnected. Within three years of an operation to remove a diseased or narrowed intestine, more than 80% of people have a recurrence if they aren't placed on treatment after their surgery.

This isn't a reason to avoid surgery if surgery will make you better. But it's important to create a well-thought-out treatment plan for after the operation that focuses on preventing a recurrence. Researchers are working on treatment strategies to help keep Crohn's disease from coming back, but right now, that's not possible in everyone.

It's also important to remember that there are different definitions of "recurrence." For some doctors, it's when the disease can be seen with an endoscope or on an X-ray even though the person with Crohn's disease has no symptoms. Other doctors define a recurrence as when symptoms develop. And still others don't believe the disease has recurred until a patient needs another operation.

An upside to surgery is that medications that may not have worked before your operation may work after your surgery.

That's because after surgery, you're essentially starting over with a clean slate that medications can maintain rather than fighting an uphill battle against existing inflammation.

TYPES OF SURGERY

The most common type of surgery for IBD is what's called a resection. This means that a part of the digestive tract is removed. This is done when disease doesn't respond to medicines, when cancer is found, or when the intestine has developed a hole (perforation).

Surgeons are learning new techniques to minimize the amount of intestine that's removed and to prevent complications and long hospital stays. The decision of how much intestine to remove is based on information gathered from X-rays, colonoscopies and biopsies. What the surgeon observes during the operation is another important factor; the surgeon can actually see and feel whether the intestine is healthy.

This type of surgery — a resection or removal of the entire colon — is increasingly being performed laparoscopically. Laparoscopic surgery results in smaller surgical scars, less postoperative pain, and shorter hospital stays.

Another technique, called stricturoplasty, may be used to limit the amount of intestine removed. With this procedure, the intestine is surgically cut and opened. This type of surgery is most often performed when there's narrowing

John had been experiencing abdominal pain for a couple of days. The pain was much worse than the frequent twinges he had experienced over the past 10 years or so. John thought it was probably something he'd eaten, because the pain was similar to what he often felt after eating a big salad or an ear of corn. The pain continued to worsen and he started running a fever that would come and go, so he went to the emergency department at his local hospital. A CT scan showed scarring of the last few inches of his small intestine, so much so that there was hardly any opening left for food to pass into the colon. Above the narrowing, the intestine was stretched (dilated) and contained food waste that was just sitting there. John quickly found himself headed to surgery to have the narrowed portion of his intestine removed. During the operation, the surgeon saw chronic inflammation associated with Crohn's disease. After surgery, John had no more pain when he ate. He realized that he'd been putting up with the discomfort for a long time, not knowing there was something wrong with his small intestine.

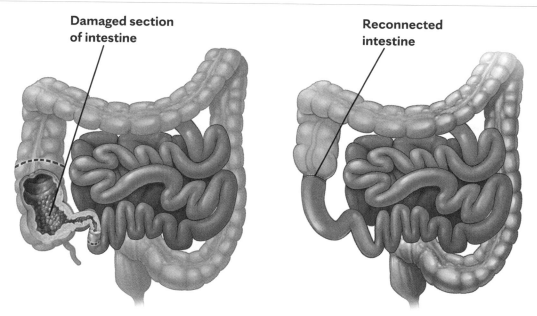

Damaged section of intestine

Reconnected intestine

With resection, the damaged portion of the intestine — small intestine or large intestine — is removed and healthy sections are reconnected.

(stricture) of the intestine. If the surgeon can open up the intestine and make it usable, it doesn't need to be removed. This surgery is often performed by colorectal surgeons who have more experience with the procedure.

Stricturoplasty is sort of like when a heart specialist performs an angioplasty. The blood vessel around the heart is stretched open and cleared of the cholesterol buildup, which avoids the need for bypass surgery. In some cases, a gastroenterologist can use a balloon to open a small narrowing (stricture) in the intestines. However, the procedure may need to be repeated several times to keep the intestine open, and it works best when there's a short narrowing of the intestines.

How long you stay in the hospital after surgery depends on the procedure you have and how sick you are before undergoing the operation.

Transplant surgery: A possibility?

The small intestine is an essential organ for sustaining life, and it is possible to transplant it. However, this type of surgery is rare and only a few medical centers in the United States are performing it. This is because intestinal transplant surgery poses many complications, and donor small intestines are difficult to come by. Also, few people are candidates for a small intestine transplant.

The reasons that someone might have transplant surgery are because:

- They've had so many operations they have hardly any intestine left.
- They have so many narrowings (strictures) that the intestine is essentially unusable.
- Their disease doesn't respond to any available medical therapy.
- They can't be on intravenous feeding because they've developed complications from it.

There's been little research on large intestine transplant surgery. Don't expect it to be a standard therapy anytime soon. Perhaps stem cell research may someday enable scientists to grow new colons. To date, however, no such research is taking place in stem cell laboratories.

SURGERY FOR ULCERATIVE COLITIS

Surgery for ulcerative colitis involves removing the colon. It's important to understand that the entire colon is removed, even if some of it is normal.

People will often ask, "How come I need to have all my colon taken out if it's just the last part that's diseased?" Many years ago, surgeons tried to remove only the affected parts and sew the remaining healthy colon to the anus. This didn't work, and patients ended up undergoing multiple surgeries with the same eventual outcome — removing the entire colon.

Imagine trying to sew a handkerchief (healthy bowel) around the top of a soda bottle (the anal canal). The kerchief is flexible and can be scrunched up, but the top of the soda bottle is fixed and stiff.

IBD SURGICAL TERMS

Colectomy. Removal of the colon.

Dysplasia. Precancerous stage in which cells have become abnormal and are likely to become cancerous.

Ileal pouch anal anastomosis. Standard operation for ulcerative colitis, in which the colon is removed.

J pouch. Shape of the pouch constructed from the small intestine used in an ileal pouch procedure.

Ostomy. Any external opening from an organ to the skin.

Resection. Removal of a section of intestine.

Stricturoplasty. The surgical opening of a narrowing in the intestine, rather than removing the segment.

Thrombosis. Blood clot.

Total parenteral nutrition. Nutritional support administered via a large vein.

Toxic megacolon. A complication of ulcerative colitis in which the colon becomes extremely dilated.

The anal canal is like that within the body. It's very difficult to figure out how to neatly cinch together all the edges of the kerchief around the top of the bottle without having uneven edges. Then, imagine trying to fill the kerchief with water and have it flow into the bottle without leaking. Impossible! That's what it's like if you try to attach the right side of the colon to the anal canal.

Surgical removal of the colon is a big, important decision to make. Sometimes, colon surgery is absolutely the right thing to do. This is often the case if you have:
- Medically resistant disease.
- Toxic megacolon.
- Cancer or precancer (dysplasia) of the colon.
- A hole in the colon (perforation).
- Bleeding that doesn't stop (hemorrhage).

If you've run out of medication options and you're not getting healthier, having your colon removed is a logical next step.

In rare cases, the colon remains so inflamed that the wall becomes dangerously thin, and the colon basically stops working. When that happens, material collects, leading to distension of the colon (a very painful condition) and fever. This is aptly called toxic megacolon because the colon has become a fully filled, inflamed poison center that needs to be removed right away. Because its walls aren't strong, the colon can perforate.

Luckily, this doesn't occur often anymore because physicians are better at determining when a colon is very sick and a person is at risk of toxic megacolon. Aggressive medical treatment is the way to prevent both toxic megacolon and severe bleeding (hemorrhage) from developing.

Colon removal

In the past, when the colon was removed, people had to live with an external bag that collected stool (ostomy). Today, the standard procedure for colon removal is an ileal pouch anal anastomosis (IPAA), also known as a J-pouch procedure. With this surgery, you don't need an ostomy bag. Eventually, you'll be able to move your bowels pretty much like anyone else and sit on the toilet when you have the sensation of needing to go.

There are only a few reasons why you might not be a candidate for this proce-

dure, so make sure to get a second opinion if you're told that you can't have it. Those reasons include the following:

- A deformed anal canal that wouldn't tolerate a connection.
- A weakened anal sphincter, which can develop as a consequence of multiple vaginal deliveries or injury to the sphincter during childbirth.
- A small intestine that's too short to allow for a pouch to be built and connected to the anal canal.
- An unhealthy final segment of the small intestine (terminal ileum).
- A history of abdominal surgeries that makes it difficult for a surgeon to safely construct a pouch and attach it to the anal canal.

The J-pouch procedure is performed in stages to allow for proper healing at each step. The first stage is to remove the colon. The surgeon creates a temporary opening (stoma) for an ileostomy that will collect digested food coming from the small intestine. Because this is a relatively simple and straightforward surgery, it can be performed by a general surgeon. If you need to have this first stage done on an emergency basis, you don't have to resort to a permanent bag just because there's no J-pouch specialist available at the time.

The next stages require a surgeon experienced in J-pouch procedures, such as a colorectal surgeon. In the second stage, a surgeon constructs a pouch from the end of your small intestine. This pouch will serve as storage for digested food. Its job is no longer to digest or process food, like it was before. In stage three, the surgeon connects the pouch to the anal canal of the rectum and removes the stoma. Sometimes these procedures may be performed in two steps. Doing it in steps allows for healing and produces the best long-term outcomes.

The J pouch functions as a reservoir, which enables you to evacuate stool (defecate). You'll have bowel movements more often than most people — six to seven times per day — but with control. The pouch is made from your small intestine and connected directly to your anal canal, which is why it's so important to make sure that the small intestine (terminal ileum) is healthy before proceeding. If there's evidence of significant inflammation in the small intestine, you may not be able to have this surgery.

The goal is for you to enjoy a better quality of life, similar to a person without IBD. The entire surgical process takes anywhere from four to 12 months. The timing depends on three things: your health at the time of the first surgery; how many steroids you're taking at the time of your surgery or the total amount you've taken over the course of your IBD, which may delay wound healing; and personal situations that make timing of the surgeries feasible, such as job considerations, family obligations and vacation plans.

In a procedure called ileoanal anastomosis, a surgeon removes the colon and innermost lining of the rectum, creates a J-shaped pouch out of the last section of the small intestine (ileum) and then reattaches the pouch near the anal sphincter. Leaving the anal sphincter and rectal muscles intact allows near-normal passage of stool.

Issues with pouches

Pouches generally perform well but may require follow-up surgery to make changes or fix problems, especially among individuals initially thought to have ulcerative colitis but later determined to have Crohn's disease. It's important for a doctor to check a pouch intermittently with a scope to make sure that it appears healthy.

Short-term complications of J-pouch surgery include leaking from the connection between the small intestine and the anal canal, diarrhea, anal leakage and obstruction from swelling or scar tissue.

Leakage

If there's a leak at the connection, you'll have pain and fever, and blood tests will signal an infection. On a CT scan, doctors will see fluid within the pelvis outside the pouch. If this occurs, the surgeon may perform an ileostomy procedure to divert the pouch temporarily and allow for healing. Diarrhea and leakage usually get better with time and adjustment to the pouch.

The frequency of leaks at suture sites is no higher in older adults than in younger individuals. But because older adults can have more cardiac and respiratory complications and require a longer hospital stay, all of this has to be taken into consideration when deciding whether to perform J-pouch surgery.

Obstruction

Swelling of the intestine from the surgery itself or scar tissue (adhesions) can make the bowel kink, causing an obstruction. Signs of obstruction include nausea, vomiting, abdominal pain, and little if any output from the pouch. Obstruction is treated with bowel rest and time. However, if the kinking persists, you'll need another operation to cut away the scar tissue. This isn't a sign that the disease has come back; rather, it's your body's reaction to the surgery itself.

Bleeding and cuffitis

Bleeding can occur from the tiny amount of rectal tissue that's usually left behind as the surgeon attaches the pouch to the anal canal. This tissue is often referred to as a cuff, and when it becomes inflamed,

the condition is known as cuffitis. The condition is usually treated with anti-inflammatory suppositories. Only in severe cases does a surgeon have to revise the pouch and remove the cuff of rectal tissue. This doesn't necessarily mean the pouch has to be removed, but it can change the way it works, including more bowel movements and some urgency.

Inflammation of the pouch

Longer-term complications may include inflammation of the pouch (pouchitis). About half of all people with a J-pouch experience at least one bout of pouchitis. The condition is easily treated with antibiotics. Symptoms include increased frequency of bowel movements, urgency, cramps and bleeding. In a few people, pouchitis can become more difficult to treat, requiring long-term antibiotics to keep the pouch healthy.

One study found that starting a certain formulation of probiotics (called VSL#3) right after surgery may prevent pouchitis. However, because not everyone gets pouchitis, this isn't a standard treatment. Probiotics aren't harmful unless they're taken in really large amounts, increasing the risk of fungal infections. However, probiotics are expensive and have to be taken every day, so it's up to you whether to use them.

Another cause of pouchitis may be Crohn's disease. As much as doctors try to make sure that they have the correct diagnosis before surgery, sometimes they can't be 100% certain. Chronic problems with the pouch, particularly if there's inflammation of the small intestine above it, suggest the culprit is Crohn's disease. All isn't lost if this is the case. The problem can be treated medically with therapies for Crohn's disease.

Some people who have Crohn's disease in the colon but have a normal small intestine may undergo surgery to remove part or all of the colon (colectomy), which includes creation of what's called a Hartmann's pouch. This is done with the understanding that if Crohn's develops in the pouch or small intestine, the person will need to begin treatment for Crohn's disease.

Weighing the benefits and potential drawbacks

Learning about the possible complications of a pouch may cause you to rethink

having the procedure, but studies show that people with pouches have just as good, if not better, quality of life than people with an intact but sick colon. Among other things, they don't have to worry about side effects of medications, and they can go to work and participate in activities without always having to be aware of where the nearest bathroom is. In addition, with the advent of laparoscopic techniques, surgical scars are smaller and cosmetic issues are minimal.

SURGERY FOR CROHN'S DISEASE

Nearly half of people with Crohn's disease need an operation at some point in their lives to manage their disease. As newer medications are developed and utilized, need for surgery has decreased. Among individuals with Crohn's disease, the most common surgeries are those to remove a section of diseased intestine in

---

ALTERNATIVE TO A J POUCH

On occasion, a different type of surgery may be performed than the standard J-pouch procedure: The small intestine is attached to the rectum and no internal pouch or stoma is created. This is generally performed if dysplasia that doesn't involve the rectum is present in the colon and the rectum isn't inflamed.

This procedure is performed in very special circumstances as just described or when a young woman is planning a pregnancy in the future (see Chapter 12). Keeping the rectum intact prevents scar tissue from forming in the pelvis. Scar tissue is often the culprit when women who've undergone J-pouch surgery later have issues with fertility.

the small or large intestine (resection) or to fix a perforation or drain an abscess.

How do you know when you need surgery?
- You aren't responding to therapy with medications, and you're getting sicker.
- You've developed a narrowing of the intestine, perhaps from a buildup of scar tissue, that's obstructing the flow of digested food.
- You have adhesions — scar tissue where damaged intestine is incorrectly healing together — that are pulling or kinking the digestive tract and causing obstruction.
- Inflammation has eaten through the intestinal wall and caused a perforation.
- You have an abscess that won't heal on its own.
- You have dysplasia or cancer.
- You have a hemorrhage that requires emergency resection. Fortunately, this is extremely rare.

Resection

In this surgery, a damaged section of the digestive tract is removed, and the healthy segments reconnected. Sometimes, more than one section may be removed during surgery. Resection is a generic term that surgeons use to describe what they do.

Fixing perforation or abscess

Crohn's disease involves inflammation of all the layers of the intestinal wall, and when the inflammation spans the entire wall, the intestine can spring a leak. This is known as a perforation, which is basically a hole or tear. Perforations can lead to swollen areas containing pus (abscesses) when stool and bacteria leak out of the bowel and into adjacent tissues and organs. As you might guess, this causes infection.

Symptoms of a perforation depend on how big the hole is. Sudden abdominal pain, fever, nausea and vomiting are all common symptoms of a perforation. An abscess may stay hidden for a while, depending on where it develops. The abdominal cavity can accommodate an abscess for a few days before symptoms may come to your attention. Low-grade fever, vague pain or even pain when straightening a leg are all symptoms of an abscess. If the abscess is positioned near the abdominal muscles that help keep your body upright or your leg straight, these may be your only symptoms. Sometimes, abscesses are only found when a CT scan is performed.

In Crohn's disease, if the perforation is small enough, medication sometimes may help it heal. Antibiotics to fight the infection and biologic and immunosuppressant medications to stop the inflammation may work together to promote healing.

Similar to repairing a leaky pipe in the basement, the first attempt to fix the problem may be to patch it or put duct tape over the leak. But when the water comes out around the patch job, the next step usually is replacement of the pipe. With a small perforation, if medication doesn't work, the next step generally is surgery to remove the damaged portion of intestine and reconnect the healthy segments.

Treating anal fistulas

Another problem that can occur in Crohn's disease is formation of an abnormal connection (fistula) in the anal area. Because the inflammation can burrow through all layers of the bowel and rectal wall, breakdown can occur around the anal canal. A fistula may start as some pain around the anal canal and a sensation of pressure. This may even lead to a feeling of fluid draining, which may be blood, stool or pus. If the fistula is small enough, sitting in a warm bath can help relieve the pressure and allow the area to drain.

Sometimes, pus can build up in an anal fistula that requires surgery to drain the area. During the procedure, a surgeon may place a temporary drain to help evacuate all the pus. A surgeon also may place a seton in the fistula tract to allow it to drain freely so that an abscess can't form. A seton is a rubber band that is sewn into place as a temporary measure while other therapies help heal the inflammation and allow the fistula to close. Sometimes setons are adjusted, particularly for large fistulas that take longer to heal. A surgeon will adjust the seton as the fistula tract gets smaller. This process doesn't hurt, as the band is simply running through the area. Unless the tract completely closes, healing tissue doesn't adhere to it. Complete closure is

rare in the time frame in which most people have a seton in place. Setons can stay in place for long periods (months to years) if a fistula proves to be especially resistant to closing. Because it prevents abscesses from recurring, it's not removed until the area is no longer inflamed and the fistula is healed enough to no longer be at risk for formation of an abscess. A seton can be removed in the office; it's pulled out just like stitches.

Hemorrhoids and skin tags

Large hemorrhoids or skin tags around the anal canal are a common complaint in people with Crohn's disease. Skin tags usually aren't felt unless they are swollen, and usually it takes an experienced pair of eyes to tell the difference between skin tags and hemorrhoids. Skin tags are benign extra growths of anal tissue, whereas hemorrhoids are swollen blood vessels in the anal canal. Some people have both, which makes the situation more confusing. Treatment includes topical creams for discomfort, medications to control diarrhea and treatment of the underlying Crohn's disease.

External hemorrhoids are found around the outside of the anal canal and can be confused for skin tags. Internal hemorrhoids aren't visible with the naked eye and aren't felt upon physical exam unless they're very swollen. Either kind can be particularly bothersome when you're dealing with diarrhea. The irritation of loose and watery stool and associated wiping can cause pain, swelling and bleeding.

When hemorrhoids are removed in people with Crohn's disease, there's a higher rate of complications, such as scarring, bleeding and infection. Therefore, surgery usually isn't recommended. If you're contemplating hemorrhoid surgery, it's recommended that you discuss the procedure and potential complications with an experienced colorectal surgeon who understands Crohn's disease.

POSTOPERATIVE COMPLICATIONS

All surgery for Crohn's disease carries with it some risk. Some risks are related to undergoing surgery in general. Others are related to the effect on the bowels specifically.

Ileus

Ileus is the term used when the intestines remain "asleep" after anesthesia, and they don't regain function quickly. We don't know why it takes longer for some people's bowels to wake up and start moving. Eventually things do start moving, but on rare occasions it can take close to 30 days for this to occur. Typically, the bowels wake up within three to five days.

Your risk of ileus may be greater if:
- Your surgery is very involved or complicated and requires significant manipulation of the intestines.
- You were taking narcotics before surgery, slowing movement of food through the digestive tract.

- You're taking a large amount of narcotics after surgery for pain control.
- It takes a long time to complete your surgery.
- You're in poor general health.

Actions thought to help get the bowels moving again after surgery include walking, deep breathing, sucking on hard candy and, for some people, chewing gum.

Blood clots

Manipulation of the intestines, not moving much after surgery and use of intravenous catheters can cause blood to pool in the veins and form blood clots. This is known as thrombosis. Clots in the large veins of the abdomen can cause pain and loss of blood flow to the intestines, interfering with healing. Clots in the legs can cause pain, swelling and redness, and they can migrate from the legs to the lungs, causing a condition called pulmonary embolism, which is life-threatening.

People with IBD are at greater risk for blood clot formation than the rest of the population, especially if the disease is very active. It's an important complication that doctors need to monitor for after an operation. IBD patients who undergo surgery are commonly treated with a blood thinner for up to 30 days after surgery to lower their risk of developing blood clots.

To help awaken your bowels and keep your blood flowing, it's important that you get up and move as quickly as you can after surgery. The sooner you can walk, the better. Even just sitting up and dangling your legs at the side of the bed or getting up to sit in a chair are important steps in your recovery. Taking slow, deep breaths to fill your lungs with air is also important.

Bowel obstruction

Soon after abdominal surgery, scar tissue begins to form. Sometimes, scar tissue grows so that it connects one section of your intestines to another loop of bowel or to the abdominal wall. This scar tissue, known as an adhesion, often causes no problems. But sometimes the bowel will kink where scar tissue develops, creating an obstruction. This isn't due to Crohn's; it's a mechanical plumbing problem.

Obstruction is part of the natural process of healing and doesn't happen more often in people with Crohn's disease than in the general population. An obstruction may cause nausea, vomiting and abdominal pain; it may seem just like a disease flare, except that you'll also stop passing stool or gas.

Obstructions are usually treated by resting the intestines and sometimes by inserting a tube through the nose into the stomach (NG tube) to decompress trapped air and fluid. In instances when the obstruction doesn't undo itself, surgery is required to unkink the bowel and cut away the scar tissue responsible for the kinking.

Wound infection

If you're taking steroids and need to have surgery, you're at higher risk of poor wound healing and the development of infection. Steroids cause thinning of the skin and blood vessels, which makes them more sensitive to manipulation and damage, even with minimal manipulation.

Abscess

An abscess may form as the result of a wound infection or a new infection at the site where the intestines were surgically connected. Antibiotics may be able to control the infection. However, depending on the size of the abscess and its location, the area may need to be drained.

Drainage of an abscess is most often performed by a radiologist. After numbing the area, the radiologist uses X-ray guidance to place a needle and drain the collection of pus. On rare occasions surgery may be necessary to drain an abscess.

Anastomotic leak

There are several reasons why the location where the intestines are reconnected may come apart, including too much tension on the connection, poor healing, infection or remaining (residual) active disease. An anastomotic leak may cause pain and fever, and an abscess may form. It can be treated but may require another operation.

Anastomotic ischemia

In this condition there's poor blood flow to the surgical site. If the reconnection between two pieces of bowel is pulled too tight, the area doesn't receive enough blood flow, damaging the intestines and causing bleeding. This is different from the ulceration in active Crohn's disease.

Acute narcotic withdrawal

If you were taking large doses of narcotics before the surgery, you may not get the same amount after surgery. This narcotic withdrawal can result in worsening pain, nausea, vomiting and even personality changes and hallucinations. Minimizing usage of narcotics before the surgery and being honest with your doctor about the amount you take can help you avoid such a complication.

Acute steroid withdrawal

If you were taking high doses of steroids before surgery, you may suffer withdrawal if you don't receive the same amount intravenously while you're recovering. Sleep and personality changes and electrolyte imbalances can occur in this situation. Fortunately, surgeons are specially trained to follow protocols for steroid dosing during and after surgery.

Diarrhea

Diarrhea can happen from the loss of absorptive surface when part or all of the bowel has been removed or when a blockage is corrected. Often, intervention is necessary, but sometimes diarrhea resolves on its own within a few days or weeks.

Long-term complications in the small intestine

When some or most of your small intestine is removed, predictable problems occur. First, you may develop bile acid diarrhea. Bile is released by the liver to help you digest fat. But it's typically absorbed by the small intestine before digested food reaches the colon. When too much of the small intestine is removed, some bile acid may enter the colon. Bile irritates the lining of the colon, which responds by producing a watery diarrhea. Medications like cholestyramine (see Chapter 6) can help. They bind bile together so that it doesn't reach the colon.

You may experience nutritional losses. The only place in the body that can absorb vitamin B-12 from food is the terminal ileum. B-12 is needed for almost every bodily function. In Crohn's disease, when the terminal ileum is inflamed or removed, vitamin B-12 can no longer be absorbed from your diet. In this situation, taking vitamin B-12 pills typically isn't helpful. You need to get the vitamin by way of monthly shots or with a special nasal spray.

Folate is another nutrient that can become depleted. Make sure that your levels are monitored after surgery to check for deficiencies. You can learn more about nutrition in Chapter 10.

Finally, short bowel syndrome is a condition that occurs in a small number of people with Crohn's disease. Normally, a person has about 500 to 600 centimeters of small intestine. When you have only 100 or fewer centimeters left, you aren't able to absorb the water and nutrients you need to survive. Risk of dehydration and complications from vitamin deficiencies is high and requires monitoring by a nutrition specialist. Most people require intravenous support with total parenteral nutrition (TPN), a method of feeding that bypasses the gastrointestinal tract.

How do you know if you have short bowel syndrome? An X-ray can measure the approximate length of your small intestine. There are no special symptoms associated with a short bowel because the diarrhea and vitamin deficiencies associated with short bowel syndrome can occur for other reasons.

STOMAS

If you have IBD, it's important that you understand stomas. A stoma is an opening in the body. Some are natural, such as the mouth, nose and anus. Some are surgically created.

Ileostomy

There are several different kinds of surgically created stomas. The most common is an ileostomy, which is an opening from the ileum in the small intestine to the abdominal wall. Output from this type of stoma is semiliquid waste, as well as gas. Because this waste doesn't interact with any bacteria, it has much less odor than regular stool. You need to empty the ileostomy bag frequently because it fills with liquid multiple times a day. It's easy to become dehydrated, and you might not realize that you have to replace the fluid that comes out of the stoma each day.

Jejunostomy

Another type of pouch is a jejunostomy, which originates from the central portion of the small intestine. This fluid contains a lot of electrolytes, and management of this stoma is the most difficult. Fortunately, this type of stoma is uncommon. It occurs when so much of the ileum is diseased that it has to be bypassed.

Colostomy

A colostomy comes off the colon; however, this is the term people commonly use to describe any form of stoma with a bag. A colostomy is used when someone with Crohn's disease has a damaged colon that can't be sewn back together. In this case, the waste is stool, which may have an odor. With this stoma, you don't have to empty the bag as frequently. This kind of surgery is generally less common in people with IBD and more common with other conditions that occur in older patients, such as colon cancer and diverticulitis.

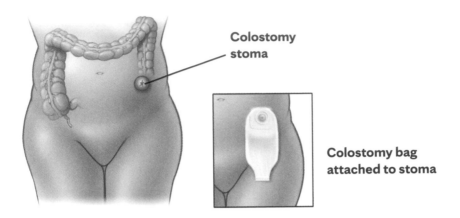

Colostomy stoma

Colostomy bag attached to stoma

A colostomy diverts stool from inside the colon to a bag outside of the body.

Continent ostomy

This type of surgery is performed by only a few surgeons around the country. A pouch is made from the small intestine, but the pouch isn't attached to the anal canal; instead, it exits the body on the anterior abdominal wall in the right lower quadrant. An external nipple is catheterized on a regular basis throughout the day to drain out the contents of the pouch. The advantage of this surgery is that you don't wear an external bag.

This surgery is highly specialized and can lead to a lot of complications. That is why it isn't the preferred surgery for anyone who needs to have their entire colon removed.

Stoma care

If you need a stoma, you'll get to know a wound care nurse, who is specially trained in the care and education of patients with stomas of all kinds. These nurses are usually affiliated with a hospital, but some surgeons have them in their private practices. If you have the opportunity, before having any surgery after which you might possibly end up with an ostomy, be sure to meet with a stoma nurse to be evaluated for the best

OTHER SURGERIES

If you need surgery for another condition, it's important to talk to the medical team so they are fully aware of your IBD and the medications you take. Make sure you inquire about which medications you may have to stop taking before the surgery and when you can start taking them again. If you're on steroids, make sure that your surgeon knows this, as you may need extra steroids during the operation.

location to place the stoma. The nurse will mark this site so that the surgeon knows exactly where the best fit will be.

Generally, a stoma is located under the belt line so that clothes or a belt won't rub on the stoma and cause trauma. Even in emergency situations, there's time for a stoma nurse to mark your abdomen for a reasonable site for a stoma; if you're able, make sure you ask about seeing a stoma nurse before emergency surgery.

Following surgery, a stoma nurse will teach you how to care for your stoma. You'll need follow-up visits to make sure that the appliance holding the bag in place has a good fit and that your skin underneath the adhesive isn't damaged. When the adhesive seal or appliance is loose, waste material can leak and damage the skin. If you gain or lose a significant amount of weight, the stoma and its outer appliance may change shape or lose its original fitting and should be reevaluated.

To sum up, surgery offers an opportunity to improve your health, but it should only happen in the right circumstances and be performed by the right surgeon. If you're very ill and have had troubles with medication, you're more likely to experience complications from surgery. Also, bear in mind that surgery generally isn't reversible. If you can, discuss your options in detail before you decide, and seek out a second opinion if it will help you feel more comfortable about your decision. Your surgeon should work closely with your other care providers to help you achieve the best health outcome.

The food fight: What can you eat?

10

Of the many and varied challenges people with IBD face, figuring out how and what to eat may be the most frustrating. More time is spent discussing diet than any other topic.

Before you began experiencing symptoms, it was reasonable for you to assume that following recommended dietary guidelines would successfully guide your body toward good health. You also may have found great pleasure in eating. Being diagnosed with IBD seemed to change everything and present you with a range of challenges. The modified dietary guidelines discussed in this chapter will help you to get all the nutrition your body needs and to make some peace with food.

We all know what it's like to eat food that doesn't agree with us. A common re-sponse is to avoid that food in the future and eat something else. You might reasonably conclude that a similar approach will work with IBD — when your GI tract is hurting, eating different foods will make you feel better. This is partly true, but the solution is not that simple. This chapter will show you how to use what you eat to better manage your disease.

A NUTRITIONAL CHALLENGE

If you broke your leg, you could find a way to get around without using that leg until it healed. That's not the case if you have a heart attack. You need to take special steps to repair your heart and to keep from having another heart attack, all the while depending on your heart to continue to beat. The same is true with IBD. Your primary organ for digesting and absorbing food is damaged. It functions, but sometimes not very well. Because your gut provides your body with the nutrients you need to survive, it needs to function while it's healing.

There are several reasons why your body may not receive all the nutrients it needs when living with IBD. During a flare, for example, a portion of your gut's lining is inflamed, which may reduce its ability to adequately absorb nutrients. Certain medications used to treat IBD make it challenging for your body to store and use certain nutrients, causing a deficiency. If you avoid certain foods to help prevent a flare, you may be missing out on necessary nutrients. Recent surgery may reduce your ability to absorb food effectively.

Nutrients are the vital ingredients in food that keep our bodies functioning. While healing from an IBD flare, your need for nutrients becomes greater. This is because a flare may increase the loss of the intestinal lining, which needs to be replaced. In addition to needing additional nutrients to help create new tissue, the inflammation associated with IBD raises your metabolic rate. That means that you're burning calories faster than when you aren't experiencing a flare.

Your metabolic rate is the rate at which your body's "engine" runs. Energy from the food we eat is converted into a form of energy that your body can use to perform its many functions. Much like a car's engine needs fuel, oil and other

fluids, the human body needs calories and nutrients to operate. Couple your body's changes in metabolism and absorption with the difficulty in eating that comes with an IBD flare, and you can see how meeting your nutritional needs can be challenging.

NUTRITION 101: WHAT EVERY BODY NEEDS

Humans need six essential nutrients to survive: carbohydrates, proteins, fats, vitamins, minerals and water. The fact that our bodies can't make many of these in sufficient amounts is the reason they're called essential. We need to obtain the nutrients from our environment in order to function.

Carbohydrates, proteins and fats — known in the nutrition world as macronutrients — provide the calories that we use daily and are needed in large enough quantities to be measured in grams or ounces. Vitamins and minerals are necessary only in very small amounts, hundredths or even millionths of a gram. They're called micronutrients. Micronutrients contain no calories but are vital to energy metabolism.

Finally, we need water, or liquids that contain water, most of all. Water plays a role in the proper functioning of nearly all our body's systems.

Most foods are combinations of carbohydrates, protein and fat and also contain various combinations of vitamins, minerals and water.

Carbohydrates

In this book, the term *carbohydrate* refers to the chemical compound (nutrient) in foods, not to the more common word denoting carbohydrate-containing foods such as potatoes, bread and rice.

Generally speaking, carbohydrates are foods composed of sugars, starches, cellulose and gums. They're the body's most preferred source of energy and a source of one of the most vital nutrients in IBD management: fiber. Carbohydrates mostly provide energy (calories) and fiber, which are found in varying quantities in grains, fruit, milk, vegetables and nuts.

You get very few calories from the fiber component of carbohydrates because the fiber is not fully absorbed. However, fiber plays a role in IBD management that's important to understand. This is addressed beginning on page 131.

There are no carbohydrates in meat or most fat-containing foods unless they're added during food preparation, which is why low-carb diets rely on a heavy intake of meat and fat.

Most foods categorized as carbohydrates contain vitamins and a few minerals. Many nutrition experts agree that in a healthy, well-balanced diet, between half and three-quarters of recommended foods are fiber-rich carbohydrates.

With fiber the key word is *whole*. Generally, the less refined the food the better it is for you. Whole grains are higher in fiber and nutrients.

Proteins

Proteins are found primarily in meat (including fish and poultry), eggs, milk and milk products, beans and nuts. In addition, most starches and vegetables contain a few grams of protein. Our bodies require quite a lot of protein, somewhere in the range of 12% to 30% of our daily intake of food.

Proteins do a lot! Protein provides the structural components of our bodies. Proteins in the form of enzymes and hormones and in genetic information (DNA, RNA) carry information throughout our bodies. Proteins tell our cells and organs how to assemble and disassemble themselves and what actions they should perform. The Greek root of the word *protein*, *proteus*, means the ability to assume different forms and implies that they come in many shapes and take on many different roles.

Fats

Fats add more than just flavor and texture to food. Dietary fats provide large amounts of energy and are necessary to the body's neurological, immune and hormone functions. Fats can be found in the form of solid fats such as butter and avocado, oils such as olive and canola oil, and waxes such as that from bees.

Like proteins, fats come in different forms: saturated, monounsaturated, polyunsaturated and trans fats. A diet high in saturated or trans fats is associated with heart disease and obesity. This is due to the inflammatory nature of these fats and the way they deposit themselves in the body's blood vessels. Healthier fats — the unsaturated types — are considered beneficial because they help turn inflammation on and off and can reduce levels of unhealthy fats in the bloodstream, thus decreasing cardiovascular disease risk.

Though it often gets a bad rap, it's important to understand that inflammation isn't something to be entirely feared. It's an important function to maintain overall health: Inflammation helps us know when we're sick and need medical attention. If you're having an allergic reaction, for example, an inflammatory response alerts you that something is wrong.

Healthy fats allow the brain to develop regular connections (a vital function in babies and young children) and to maintain those connections, especially as we age. Some vitamins can only be broken down by fat, not water. So, we need fats to get those vitamins into our tissues. Fats also control the regulation of hormones in our bodies, especially those related to appetite, metabolism and even reproduction. Finally, fats provide us with insulation to keep the body warm and help cushion our organs in case of blows and other trauma.

Polyunsaturated fats include the omega-3 and omega-6 fatty acids you may have heard about. Eicosapentaenoic acid (EPA) and docosahexaenoic acid (DHA) are omega-3 fatty acids found in fish oil, which may be beneficial to individuals with IBD. Omega-3 fatty acids have anti-inflammatory properties and may decrease active inflammation.

Trials performed in Europe indicated that omega-3 supplements can treat the active symptoms of Crohn's disease. Unfortunately, the formulation of fish oil used in those trials isn't available in the United States and is equivalent to eating 2 to 3 pounds of fish per day. Two other studies, which used omega-3 supplements after surgery to prevent recurrence of Crohn's disease, were unable to replicate this finding. So, it's unclear how we should use omega-3 in the treatment of Crohn's disease, especially when and at what dose.

Despite these uncertain findings, supplementing your diet with omega-3s may provide an anti-inflammatory benefit and assist in overall management of IBD. The recommended daily dose of omega-3s depends on the formulation and other medications that you may be taking. That's because omega-3s can interfere with certain medications. It's best to ask your health care provider about the appropriate dose and what form would best suit you.

Following a Mediterranean-style diet, including two servings of fish per week along with ample amounts of olive oil, is believed to be beneficial for patients with IBD. On the other hand, omega-6 fatty acids (safflower oil, corn oil, walnuts) have properties that promote inflammation and may be best avoided.

Keep in mind the calories in fat can add up quickly — a gram of dietary fat contains more than twice as many calories as a gram of carbohydrate or protein. Historically, fats have gained a bad reputation because their high calorie levels often are associated with weight gain and inflammation. But they play an important role in overall health and thus deserve more respect. In a healthy diet, between 20% and 35% of calories should come from fats.

Vitamins

Survival and good health are dependent on getting 13 essential vitamins from the food we eat. These vitamins have multiple functions in our bodies and allow a variety of chemical reactions to occur. For example, vitamins help build up and repair tissues, convert food into energy and even bolster our immune system.

The B vitamins and vitamin C are water soluble and thus are absorbed and carried with the liquid in our blood. Vitamins A, D, E and K must be consumed along with fat in our food in order to be absorbed. This is because they travel attached to fat molecules in our blood to reach the cells that need them.

In the management of IBD, use of certain medications and the presence of fat malabsorption can make consuming, storing and utilizing essential vitamins challenging.

Minerals

Minerals perform a surprising number of roles. Here's just a partial list:

- Calcium is incorporated into bone, and, among other things, it helps blood to clot and our heart to beat.
- Iron combines with oxygen and carries oxygen in blood to tissues, where the oxygen is released.
- Sodium and potassium control the amount and location of water in the body. Potassium helps muscles contract, a function that's necessary for the heart to beat.
- Copper is found in enzymes that drive certain vital reactions. Copper is also a component of hormones and helps make red blood cells.

Except for a few, like calcium and magnesium, most minerals are needed in very small quantities. Most people with IBD don't have problems getting small quantities of minerals. But they often struggle to get those needed in larger quantities, such as calcium. Calcium is the most abundant mineral in our bodies and is discussed in more detail on page 137.

Water

Water and other fluids containing water that we drink do more than just quench our thirst. They're essential to life and keeping our bodies functional. Nearly all of our body systems rely on water to complete their functions. Water is responsible for things like regulating temperature, lubricating joints, dissolving minerals and nutrients and getting nutrients and oxygen to our cells.

Research on how much water and other fluids a person should drink each day is lacking, but there's a general consensus that the average person needs a minimum of 1,500 to 2,000 milliliters (50 to 64 ounces) per day to replace fluid losses associated with sweating, urination and defecation. How much you need is dependent on factors such as climate, kidney function, heart function, medications, surgical history and nutrition status.

YOUR INDIVIDUAL NUTRITION NEEDS

A great deal of research over the last 100 years has enabled major health organizations to reach fairly close agreement on the amount of carbohydrates, proteins and fats the average human needs to remain healthy. But the fact is, individual needs vary.

Your genetic makeup and your environment work together to determine how much of a particular vitamin or mineral — or even fat, carbohydrate and protein — your body needs at any particular time. For example, because of your IBD, you may need more protein when you're having or recovering from a bout of inflammation. That's because your body uses protein to repair itself.

Because IBD is a nutritionally demanding condition and the disease can lead to intermittently poor intake of necessary nutrients, it's a good idea to take a multivitamin daily, unless your health care provider tells you otherwise. You want a complete multivitamin you find tolerable.

Remember that some medications used to treat IBD can result in deficiency of

several micronutrients. For example, use of the medication cholestyramine can deplete fat-soluble vitamins, resulting in deficiencies of vitamins A, D, E and K. Use of the medication methotrexate can lead to deficiencies in folate and B vitamins.

If you need extra folic acid or iron, consider a prenatal vitamin, particularly if you're a woman in your childbearing years. Because iron supplements can cause gastrointestinal side effects, take supplements with iron only if you have a diagnosed deficiency. In some situations, patients with IBD and iron deficiency may need to receive intravenous iron replacement, which is typically given as two doses one week apart.

IBD-required modifications

When your disease is active, you may modify your diet. If it makes you feel better, you probably won't mind doing that. However, even after the inflammatory stage is over and you're feeling better again, you may find that certain foods continue to irritate your gut and cause symptoms. Understandably, you may want to continue to avoid those foods all or most of the time to prevent ongoing symptoms.

There may be foods that need to be off limits at certain times but eaten as much as you can tolerate the rest of the time. Fiber is the most obvious. During a flare you may avoid it, but once you're healed, fiber is an essential part of a healthy diet and important to IBD management. You also may want to avoid certain foods during a flare that ordinarily wouldn't bother you, such as dairy products, some herbs and spices and even hot or cold foods. You may find it's easier to tolerate smaller, more frequent meals because they're less likely to cause bowel distention and excessive gas than infrequent, larger meals.

While red meat is an excellent source of protein and iron, it is particularly high in saturated fat, is difficult to digest and can promote inflammation. The protein structure of red meat requires a lot of effort from your digestive tract to break it down for absorption. Digestion depends on the mechanical effort of your teeth (chewing), the grinding (churning) of your stomach to physically break food down, and the chemicals (enzymes and acids) found in your GI tract to chemically break it down.

Foods like red meat, with muscle fibers that are largely dense, can lead to bloating, pain, constipation and even diarrhea if the meat is too high in fat. The World Health Organization recommends that the general population limit intake of red meat, even stating that there are no known safe amounts to include in a healthy diet. With higher intakes of red meat associated with increased risk of certain bowel cancers, dietary experts had to get serious with their recommendations. The risk of cancer may be even higher in people with IBD because of chronic inflammation in the GI tract. As a result, most nutrition experts encourage people with IBD to limit or avoid red meat as much as possible.

It's important to understand that while you need to consume more protein during a flare, the body can only digest about 20 to 30 grams at any given time. If the smallest steak at a restaurant is 9 ounces, and each ounce provides an average of 7 grams of protein, this adds up to 63 grams at one meal. This, coupled with the difficult-to-digest nature of steak, could lead to unnecessary stomach distress, without much payoff. For some people, a 9-ounce steak might seem small, but it's far more than the body can handle. It's best to keep your portions to 3 to 4 ounces, targeting 21 to 28 grams per meal or snack.

You may need more dietary modifications if you have Crohn's disease than if you have ulcerative colitis. This is because tissue damage from Crohn's disease usually occurs in areas of the small intestine most involved in nutrient absorption, thereby preventing uptake of the nutrients. Also, medications used to treat Crohn's disease can cause loss of nutrients as well as increase your need for protein.

Learn to let experience be your guide. You can help keep your IBD under control by being observant of trends and connections. How good are you at paying attention to the signals that your body provides when you feel better or worse? Can you tell when you have more energy or less, or how often you're experiencing flares? These signals aren't necessarily due to nutrition, but they may be. It's a good idea to listen to your body and see if anything stands out to you. Sometimes you're the best expert!

Keeping a food diary may help you learn how your body responds to different foods. Write down the different foods you eat, when you eat them, and approximately how much you eat. If you experience symptoms, write down the time and a description of how you feel. Over time, you'll likely begin to see trends; certain foods and symptoms may occur together, one following the other. Having this information will make it easier for you to limit those foods when needed. A food diary is a good tool for effective IBD self-management.

FIBER AND RESIDUE

Almost all the nutrients in the food we consume are extracted from food waste while it's in the small intestine, where nutrients pass into the bloodstream for delivery to cells throughout the body. Remaining food waste, nearly all plant material, continues on through the gastrointestinal tract.

This plant material is what we refer to as fiber and what your grandparents probably called roughage. It's primarily the

SAMPLE FOOD DIARY

Time	Food/Amount	Symptom
8:00 a.m.	black coffee, 1 cup orange juice oatmeal with milk	
10:30	muffin	
11:30		diarrhea, cramps
1:00 p.m.	fruit smoothie	
4:00		bad diarrhea
6:00	green beans rice BBQ pork chop tossed salad	
8:00		pain, cramping
10:00	oatmeal cookie	
3:00 a.m.		explosive bm, mucus, cramps

structural parts of plants, like the cell walls, which are mostly indigestible (can't be fully broken down) carbohydrates and a small amount of lignin. Lignin is a complex organic polymer found in plant tissues.

Residue, another term you may encounter, includes not only fiber but all the contents that remain in the large intestine — other undigested food, bacteria, intestinal secretions and intestinal cells that have sloughed off as they're replaced by new cells. Sometimes a low-fiber diet is called a low-residue diet because residue acts as a stool-bulking agent, but this use can be confusing.

Think of residue like the soap residue on the shower tile; the residue in your intestines can build up and cause bloating and discomfort. This is why, historically, low-fiber or low-residue diets were recommended for people with IBD. Low-fiber diets, however, are no longer recommended unless you have a narrowing (stricture) in your intestines or you're in the midst of a flare.

Solubility and insolubility

Fiber is divided into two types: soluble and insoluble. It's one type or the other depending on whether it dissolves in water. That's a bit of an oversimplification, but it's accurate enough to build on for a broader understanding of how each kind of fiber is categorized and used by your body. The two types of fiber act somewhat differently in our bodies and perform different functions, each important to bowel health.

Fiber passes through the esophagus, stomach and small intestine unaffected by our digestive enzymes. Insoluble fiber, however, is broken into gradually smaller pieces by way of chewing, stomach acid and the rough-and-tumble churning of our stomach and intestinal contractions. Soluble fiber dissolves in the water in the gut. Although fiber isn't digested in the small intestine, it still performs useful functions in the upper digestive tract, such as slowing stomach emptying and lengthening the time it takes for sugar in a meal to be absorbed. Generally, these actions have a beneficial effect on your overall health and how you feel.

Fiber that dissolves in water produces a smooth, almost slimy slurry that moves slowly through the gut. It's similar to the texture of finely ground oatmeal after cooked in water and allowed to cool slightly. Insoluble fiber maintains its rough texture and is anything but smooth and slippery. It primarily serves to slide or scrape alongside the inner lining of the intestines and colon to keep them clean. This may sound painful and scary, but it's important for the health of your GI tract.

When it reaches the large intestine, some of the fiber is digested after all — not by digestive enzymes but by "good" bacteria that reside in the large intestine. "Good" and "bad" bacteria that reside in our intestines are what's known as our microbiome. These microbes find their way to our digestive tract mostly through our diet and environment.

Both soluble fiber and insoluble fiber absorb several times more water than their own volume, making stool bulkier, softer and easier to pass. Because of this, fiber and its residue can stretch (distend) your large intestine, which can be uncomfortable when the colon is inflamed and sensitive. Add this to the byproducts of bacterial digestion (gas and water), and you can understand why you may want to avoid too much fiber during a flare. The action that moves the fecal mass through the large intestine can hurt!

It's OK to avoid fiber for a short time to give your inflamed gut a rest, but you should do this only if necessary, and you should reintroduce fiber as soon as you're able. Remember, you have a colony of bacteria to keep alive! Even if you have to avoid it at certain times, fiber is still good for you: it's a necessary component of a healthy diet that your body needs for long-term gut health.

Gut microbiome

Did you know that prior to birth a baby's colon is completely sterile? Yes, sterile! It becomes colonized by bacteria and microbes as it travels through a mother's birth canal and later through skin-to-skin contact with parents. The types and amounts of colonic bacteria are basically a fingerprint unique to each person that exists not in the thousands but in the hundreds of trillions. Good bacteria from the body's microbiome are thought to be more than 70% responsible for its immune function.

Medical professionals around the globe are studying the microbiome to try to learn what they can about its role in chronic disease and overall bodily function. When we eat foods, specifically ones containing fiber, our microbiome uses this as a fuel source to stay alive and complete its functions in our large intestine. We provide the good bacteria with a fuel source, or food, in the form of soluble fiber. Bacteria, in turn, convert the fiber into water, gas and a magical substance called short-chain fatty acids (SCFAs) that cells in our colons use for energy. Our colons must have SCFAs to survive and stay healthy.

While there's still much to be learned about the microbiome, we do know that having a more diverse microbiome is associated with overall better bowel health. A more diverse microbiome has even been associated with a reduction in the rate of IBD. We also know that people with the widest diversity of good microbes consume the widest variety of plant-based foods, the source of fiber.

Think of the microbiome and its relationship with fiber like a colony of people, all with different food needs for survival. Some may need asparagus to live, for example, while others might need beets or even mushrooms. If you deprive the microbiome of its sources of food for extended periods of time, certain bacteria die. The result is less diverse microbes in your body. Long story short, variety is thought to be far more important than quantity. For example, eating 20 servings of green beans every week is far less likely to benefit your microbiome than eating 10 smaller servings of 10 different plant-based foods.

Fiber guidelines

The Academy of Nutrition and Dietetics recommends that adults consume a minimum of 25 to 35 grams of fiber each day and that children consume enough grams of fiber each day to equal their age plus five. Because food labels provide the amount of fiber per serving, it's easy to develop a sense of how much fiber you get from packaged foods.

You'll likely be able to eat the recommended amount of fiber when your IBD is inactive and your bowel isn't inflamed. However, some people with IBD find that eating fiber is challenging regardless of disease activity. If you're just learning how to deal with your disease, use a food diary to keep track of your fiber intake. You want to make sure that you're getting a healthy amount but also watch for trends in the activity of your disease. Try not to let yourself believe that fiber is the enemy. It does a great deal to keep cells in your intestines healthy and to prevent relapses, provided you consume it when your gut is able to deal with it.

Adding fiber

If you're recovering from a flare and your health care provider or a dietitian has instructed you to increase your fiber intake, there are a few rules of thumb to remember. The first is to increase your intake very slowly, only a few grams more each week. For example, you might try one-fourth cup of oatmeal for soluble fiber and a quarter piece of whole-wheat toast for insoluble fiber. Skip a day and do it again. Then, increase it to every day. After a week, double the amount of oatmeal and add a few small pieces of canned fruit or a half cup of a soft, thin-skinned vegetable you haven't been eating. Continue in this manner until you've reached the amount your provider or dietitian recommends.

The second rule of thumb is to drink a lot of fluid, enough to keep your urine a very pale yellow. If it's bright yellow, you may not be getting enough water. Fiber absorbs water to keep it soft and easy to pass. If enough water isn't available, you may experience severe, uncomfortable constipation.

The third rule of thumb is to not get discouraged. Try softer versions of each food first — think of it as following the preparation method. Start with cooked, stewed or even pureed versions that promote tolerance of fiber-containing foods, especially if it's been a while since you last ate them. Increase only to amounts that you can tolerate.

Remember, with microbiome diversity, the key is to consume a variety of different sources of fuel (fiber), not necessarily the largest quantity. As you're able, add less-cooked or raw fiber-rich foods.

If you're struggling with identifying which foods are good sources of fiber, consider investing in one of the many phone apps or books that list foods and their fiber contents. Some books are small enough to fit into a pocket or purse. They can be quite handy when you're unsure which choices to make.

LACTOSE INTOLERANCE

If you have Crohn's disease, your doctor may have told you to avoid lactose-containing foods, or you may have already figured out for yourself that milk and milk products cause you problems. Lactose intolerance is the inability to digest lactose, a form of sugar naturally found in milk. For many adults and almost all children, lactose is digested in the small intestine and broken down by an enzyme produced there called lactase. When this enzyme isn't produced in sufficient amounts to break down lactose, lactose intolerance occurs.

If your small intestine is inflamed or damaged, which may occur with Crohn's disease, you're less likely to produce enough lactase to digest lactose, and thus you can develop "conditional" lactose intolerance (meaning it's likely to cause you problems only during the conditions of a flare). If you have ulcerative colitis, it's less likely that you'd become lactose intolerant because the inflammation is in your colon rather than in the small intestine.

If you're lactose intolerant and drink milk or eat food with milk in it, you may experience some or all of the following symptoms: gas, bloating, loose and urgent bowel movements, cramping and pain. Lactose intolerance is generally diagnosed by matching your symptoms with what you ate or by performing what's called hydrogen breath testing. Lactose that you were unable to digest is digested by bacteria in your colon. These bacteria create byproducts, one of which is hydrogen. The extra hydrogen is carried in the bloodstream to the lungs and shows up at abnormally high levels in your breath.

If your disease is active and you're experiencing lactose intolerance, avoid drinking or eating products with lactose in them. This means totally avoiding regular or flavored milks, evaporated or condensed milk, ice cream or frozen yogurt, buttermilk, cream soups, large amounts of cheese, perhaps butter, and milk-based pudding. While yogurt, kefir and small amounts of cheese are milk products, they're relatively well tolerated by individuals with lactose intolerance. This is due to the probiotic content of yogurt and kefir that assists in the digestion of lactose and the relatively low lactose content of cheese.

Most products that contain lactose are fairly obvious. However, there are less obvious sources, such as ready-to-drink and powdered nutritional supplements. Many of these products list the lactose-containing ingredients on the label as casein (the solid part of milk), whey (the liquid part of milk), and milk solids or milk protein, so be sure to check the ingredients on food labels. Finally, you need to be aware of the truly sneaky sources of lactose: drugs and supplements that use lactose as a filler. Again, read the labels and, if you're unsure, ask your pharmacist.

Once the inflammation in your gut has subsided and you're again able to include more options in your list of tolerated foods, it may be safe for you to try reintroducing lactose into your diet. Most people with lactose intolerance can eventually tolerate somewhere between one-half and one cup of regular milk a day without unpleasant symptoms. However, don't expect or try to do this immediately after a flare.

Lactose-free milk and milk products are widely available, so people with lactose intolerance can still enjoy this excellent source of protein. Some brands that are either lactose-free or that contain lactose-digesting enzymes are Lactaid, Fairlife and Smart Balance. Look for them in the refrigerated section near the other kinds of milk and be sure to select options that are advertised as lactose-free.

Lactase enzyme pills are available over the counter at most pharmacies and in many grocery stores. You chew two or three of the pills immediately before drinking or eating foods containing lactose to enhance its absorption. The pills don't break down all the lactose, but they help. This may allow you to eat foods in which lactose is present — certain breads, sherbets or restaurant dishes with butter or cream, for example. Timing is the key to using these pills. If you take them too soon, your stomach will break down the enzymes (your stomach considers them just another protein to digest), rendering them ineffective. It's wise to carry some with you in case you find yourself faced with more lactose than you think you can handle.

Finally, there are other kinds of milk that contain no lactose. Soy, rice and almond milks can be found in most large supermarkets. They're perfectly OK for you to consume, at least in terms of lactose. However, with the exception of soy milk, they're mostly flavored water and quite low in protein and carbohydrates. Drinking a glass will not be nearly as nutritious as a glass of lactose-free milk. It's a matter of trial and error, but with patience and careful record keeping, you may find that living with lactose intolerance isn't difficult.

If you're still experiencing gas, cramping and further digestive upset after consuming lactose-free varieties of cow's milk, lactose might not be the culprit. For some people, the intact proteins in milk are too difficult to break down comfortably and can lead to symptoms similar to that of lactose intolerance. While this can result from a true cow's-milk allergy, in which cow's milk needs to be completely avoided, you might first try easier-to-digest milk-based foods. As previously discussed, yogurt and kefir may be viable options because the probiotics in them make them easier to digest.

Oral nutrition supplements with specialized processing are another possibility. For example, in 100% whey protein isolate, there is so little lactose that it can't be detected and the more difficult-to-digest casein protein has been removed. Therefore, it's a source of protein that people with IBD tend to tolerate very well. Whey protein isolate is most commonly found in clear liquid-based supplements like Ensure Clear and Isopure Protein Water and powder-based supplements like Blue Bonnet 100%

Whey Isolate. Be sure to look for products with 100% whey isolate as the only source of protein, and try to pick ones with the smallest list of ingredients. This will help ensure that you're limiting as many variables as possible that could trigger symptoms.

Common protein supplements that you may need to avoid because they contain more intact proteins and possibly intolerable amounts of lactose are identifiable as the following ingredients: milk protein, milk protein concentrate, casein protein, milk solids and whey protein concentrate.

CALCIUM: A SPECIAL PROBLEM

The absorptive lining of your small intestine — the villi — may be so damaged by inflammation due to Crohn's disease that it may not function much at all, or it may need to be surgically removed. When the lining is damaged, it's easy for you to become deficient in a number of nutrients. Calcium poses a special problem. You see, our bodies need a lot of calcium to function, and with milk being its most abundant source, consuming adequate amounts can be difficult, especially if you're avoiding it during times of intolerance.

Drugs that are used to suppress inflammation in the GI tract, such as steroids, methotrexate and cyclosporine, can cause calcium to be lost from bones, making you especially prone to osteopenia, osteoporosis and even calcium-based renal stones. Surgical alterations to your intestines can also put you at risk for calcium-based renal stones. If you're limiting dairy because of intolerance, getting adequate calcium can become tricky. Between malabsorption, reduced intake, surgical changes and calcium loss from bones, calcium deficiency may become severe. Calcium fuels many processes in your body in addition to keeping your bones strong, so it's vital to take this seriously.

Historically, people prone to kidney stones were told to avoid calcium supplements. But if you're avoiding dairy products (natural calcium), this can put you at risk for deficiency, which can actually lead to the formation of more stones. The best way to prevent this is to include adequate dairy in your diet. Most people with IBD can tolerate lactose-free dairy products, which can help meet the overall need for calcium. If you find this isn't the case for you, a calcium supplement, preferably in the form of calcium citrate, could be an option.

Calcium citrate is one of the gentler forms of supplemental calcium when taken in amounts of 500 milligrams or less, and it's readily available over the counter. Unlike other sources of artificial calcium, calcium citrate makes urine more acidic, so it's a less hospitable environment for stones to form.

If you need to take more than 500 milligrams per day of calcium because you aren't consuming enough dairy, you'll want to take your supplements throughout the day to promote tolerance. You should avoid taking them with iron supplements, because iron can inhibit the absorption of calcium. Avoiding artificial calcium is generally the safest option if you have certain types of kidney stones. Artificial calcium is commonly found in multivitamins, oral nutrition supplements (protein shakes and powders) and dairy alternatives like soy, almond and coconut milk products.

There are nondairy sources of natural calcium, such as green, leafy vegetables. However, they contain a compound called oxalate that inhibits the absorption of the calcium they contain and are often associated with other types of renal stones. They're also often high in insoluble fiber, which may be poorly tolerated during an IBD flare.

You may also need to increase your intake of vitamin D, which helps calcium to be deposited in bone. It's not unusual to be deficient in both at the same time. Under ideal conditions, people manufacture vitamin D in their skin when it's exposed to sunlight. If you live in a southern sunny climate, you're less likely to be deficient in this vitamin, but people vary in the amount of vitamin D they're able to produce from this source. Although there are some good food sources of vitamin D, it's hard to eat enough to compensate for a deficiency. Therefore, we generally recommended taking oral supplements if you need additional vitamin D.

Taking your calcium and vitamin D supplements together is a great way to enhance absorption. In adults with IBD, the current recommendations are 1,500 milligrams per day of calcium and 1,000 international units (IU) of vitamin D per day. The more you can get from food, however, the better.

TRIGGER FOODS

When you experience an IBD flare, it's easy to believe it's because of something you ate. You have gas and bloating and pain in your abdomen. It didn't hurt before you ate, so it must be the food, right? While this sounds reasonable, it's only partly correct.

Keep in mind that IBD is an inflammatory disease in which your immune system attacks your intestine. What causes a flare isn't fully understood. Certain foods — beans, for example — cause gas and bloating in most people, even people who don't have IBD. Likewise, a sudden large intake of sugar alcohols, a sugar alternative found in some candies, nutritional supplements and desserts, will often cause diarrhea. These artificial sugars attract a large amount of water to your colon and, when consumed in large quantities, have a laxative effect. Subsequent diarrhea happens to everyone who consumes them in large quantities, not just to people with IBD.

In essence, certain foods have inherent properties that determine how they're going to interact with the gastrointestinal tract. Think of it like a cut on your hand: You wouldn't pour lemon juice on the cut, right? That would make the cut hurt worse, although it won't slow healing. It's the same with the wrong food: It doesn't cause inflammation, but it can give you symptoms that make you feel worse.

When you experience abdominal pain, there's really no clear-cut way of knowing whether it was the food, your immune system or both behind your discomfort. It might be the early stages of a flare, or it might not.

A common response to having a flare after consuming a trigger food is to eliminate that food from your diet. Unfortunately, that food may not be the cause, and you've limited your diet unnecessarily. Over time, you may find that you've severely restricted your diet, even to the point of developing malnutrition.

A better approach is to keep careful records of what you eat. By reviewing what you ate over the course of several flares, you may begin to see if there are common triggers. If so, we suggest eliminating those foods for a period of maybe six to eight weeks to see if you have fewer symptoms. You can reintroduce the suspected food in small doses and see if the symptoms return.

The main thing to remember is that everyone with IBD is unique in relation to foods that seem to cause symptoms. Just because you have Crohn's disease doesn't mean that you have the same dietary intolerances as another person with the disease. A good analogy for this is perfumes. You go to the department store, and there are hundreds available. What smells good on you may not smell good on your sister or best friend, because it has to do with personal body chemistry. The same holds true for foods and diets: It isn't one size fits all.

In fact, your health care provider may tell you that if you have ulcerative colitis, it doesn't matter what you eat. What he or she means is that it's unlikely that what you eat will contribute significantly to the entire inflammatory process that's occurring.

Diet is only one part of the puzzle. Medications and surgery, when indicated, are integral to the overall treatment of IBD, along with nutrition and lifestyle therapies. While there are inherent properties in foods that may produce GI symptoms, they could occur in anyone, not just in someone with IBD. Your own experiences are the best guide for what affects you.

REACTIONS TO GLUTEN AND MORE

Celiac disease, or celiac sprue, results from an autoimmune reaction to the gluten in wheat and other grains. Celiac disease is not the same as having a food allergy. The reaction that occurs with celiac disease is different from what happens with IBD. In the case of celiac disease, nutrient-absorbing villi that line the small intestine are severely damaged; over time, nutrient deficiencies can occur as well as malnutrition. However, the symptoms of celiac disease and IBD are similar — diarrhea, gas, bloating and cramps.

The treatment for celiac disease is complete avoidance of items containing gluten, which includes most breads and products made with gluten-containing grains. Unfortunately, gluten is added to many foods and even some medications, making it difficult to avoid without being a food detective.

People with IBD sometimes feel better when they remove gluten from their diet, but that doesn't mean that they have celiac disease. When you take out such a common entity, it often means that you're eating more fresh foods and preparing meals at home rather than eating out. A return to fresh foods and homemade meals often results in a better tolerance of food.

The experience of fewer symptoms after eliminating gluten is often improperly correlated to the absence of gluten rather than decreased inflammation due to an increase in short-chain fatty acids resulting from eating more vegetables and fruits. Remember, short-chain fatty acids are the magical anti-inflammatory byproduct of fiber digestion. While going gluten-free can be an overall healthy way to eat, removing gluten doesn't cure IBD, and such a strict diet isn't necessary to improve your symptoms.

Some people wonder if they've been misdiagnosed and actually have a food allergy instead of IBD. There's certainly a lot we don't understand about the immune system and the way it interacts with the digestive tract, and it's impossible to tell someone with certainty that he or she isn't having some sort of allergic reaction to certain foods in addition to IBD.

Proving the presence of a food allergy means systematically working your way through tedious food elimination diets and carefully reintroducing individual foods to watch for a return of symptoms. A food allergy tends to be predictable once you find the culprit, because the absence of that particular food results in well-being and its reintroduction produces symptoms every time you're exposed to the food. We haven't found such a straightforward link between any one food and IBD.

With IBD affecting so many different people, each with varied diets and sources of calories, it seems unlikely that we'll find a common dietary ingredient behind the symptoms.

YOUR NEED FOR GLUTAMINE

Keeping the cells that line the intestinal tract as healthy as possible is a major goal for people with IBD. One way of doing this is to keep those cells well fed. And one of their foods of choice is an amino acid called glutamine, which has historically been of particular interest to people with IBD.

Glutamine is a major component of dietary protein. It's also the most common amino acid in the body, especially with muscle and blood. You know by now that all foods that contain calories (with the exception of alcohol) are composed of carbohydrates, fats and proteins, either separately or mixed together in different proportions and different arrangements. That seems pretty simple to remember. However, each of these main categories is itself composed of different arrangements of their own primary ingredients — sugars and starches in carbohydrates, fatty acids in fats, and amino acids in proteins. There are 21 different kinds of amino acids from which proteins can be assembled, and each performs a slightly different function.

One of the functions of glutamine is to help maintain the health of the cells that line the intestinal tract (intestinal mucosa). By keeping these cells well nourished, they can better fight off disease-causing organisms. These cells also work synergistically with short-chain fatty acids and your microbiome to prevent a leaky gut, in which molecules from food, ingested toxins or bacteria leak into the blood due to intestinal damage. There's also some evidence that the leaking of these molecules plays a role in the immune response associated with IBD. Glutamine is helpful in restoring tissue damaged during an inflammatory flare.

Fortunately, glutamine is abundant in foods that are generally well tolerated. The easiest way to get extra glutamine into your diet is to eat plenty of poultry, fish and red meat. Beans and dairy products are also rich in glutamine, but because of the high fiber content of beans and lactose intolerance associated with dairy products, you may not be able to tolerate them in ample amounts until your gut recovers. Some vegetables and fruits are also rich in this amino acid.

Glutamine can be found in powdered supplements; it's more concentrated when consumed this way. At one point, glutamine supplements were thought to

be a viable therapeutic option for people with IBD because of promising benefits in some animal studies. To date, however, there haven't been any human studies to support a beneficial role of supplemental glutamine in IBD. Therefore, it's not routinely recommended.

MALNUTRITION IN IBD

Unfortunately, it's not uncommon for people with IBD to experience malnutrition. Being malnourished doesn't necessarily mean being underweight. Malnutrition occurs when nutrient supplies that your body needs to function properly aren't consumed or stored in adequate amounts. This is most likely to happen when abdominal pain causes loss of appetite and you become afraid to eat and severely restrict your diet.

Another cause of malnutrition among people with IBD is the intestine's loss of ability to absorb nutrients and fluids. This overall reduction in the body's access to nutrients can lead to vitamin and mineral deficiencies, loss of weight and loss of body fat and muscle.

To prevent or reverse malnutrition:
- *Calories.* Eat enough calories. Most adults with IBD require 25 to 35 calories per kilogram of their body weight. If you're in a flare, you may need more.
- *Protein.* Eat enough protein. Most adults with IBD benefit from eating 1 to 1.5 grams of protein per kilogram of their body weight. Remember that 1 ounce of meat or fish = 7 grams of protein.

- *Nutritional supplement.* If you can't eat adequate amounts of healthy foods, consider an oral nutritional supplement, such as a ready-to-drink protein shake or powders added to food. A calorie-concentrated formula may be needed if you require a large number of supplemental calories per day. These concentrated liquids usually have twice as many calories per ounce as regular ones.
- *Multivitamin.* Consider vitamin and mineral supplementation, especially folic acid, vitamin D, vitamin B-12, zinc and iron.
- *Folic acid.* Taking the medications sulfasalazine or methotrexate may alter folic acid absorption and metabolism, requiring folic acid supplementation. Folic acid also protects against colon cancer.
- *Vitamin D.* An increase in disease activity can promote vitamin D deficiency and contribute to low bone mineral density and osteoporosis. In fact, a lack of vitamin D is the most common deficiency in people with Crohn's disease. Recommended dosing is 800 to 1,000 IU per day in pill or capsule form.
- *B-12.* The terminal ileum is where B-12 is absorbed. If you have disease there or your ileum has been removed, you're at increased risk for B-12 deficiency. Bacterial overgrowth also appears to increase the risk. B-12 deficiency is treated with periodic injections of 100 to 1,000 micrograms per month or 50 to 100 micrograms of sublingual forms (liquids or melts placed under the tongue). Some people need to self-administer monthly B-12 injections.

- *Zinc.* Severe diarrhea, enteric fistulas and moderate-to-severe disease activity can result in zinc deficiency. The recommended daily allowance is 15 milligrams per day, which is provided by many formulations of over-the-counter supplements. If you're found to be deficient, you may need a larger dose. This is generally prescribed for a short period of time, as zinc supplements are irritating to the GI tract, and when taken for periods longer than 14 days, they can lead to deficiency in copper.
- *Iron.* Bleeding, lack of appetite and decreased absorption all can lead to iron deficiency. It's common in IBD, particularly in ulcerative colitis, so make sure your iron levels are monitored. Recommended supplementation for deficiency is 150 to 200 milligrams of elemental iron per day, in addition to increasing your intake of iron-rich foods. Iron supplements are best absorbed when taken with a source of vitamin C. Routine iron supplementation should be avoided unless you're proven deficient, as it can lead to abdominal pain, constipation and cramping.

WHEN YOU CAN'T EAT FOOD

There may be times when you need supplemental nutrition: you're not eating enough to stay nourished, you're losing too much weight or you're not gaining the weight that you need to stay healthy. If you hear your health care providers talk about enteral nutrition, that means supplying calories directly to the GI tract.

Enteral nutrition can take the form of supplements or specialized formulas that may contain predigested or elemental nutrients so that your body doesn't have to work as hard to break them down. These nutrients can be consumed by mouth, although they're more often given via feeding tubes placed in the nose, stomach or small intestine. In addition to supplementing your eating, they may be used as your only source of nutrition when you're very sick during a severe flare.

Studies have shown that nutritional therapy using enteral products, especially in children with Crohn's disease, can result in disease remission rates quite similar to when corticosteroids are used. This is perhaps because this therapy ensures that the intestines have an adequate source of fuel to maintain the microbiome and repair the intestines. Few people want enteral nutrition as their sole source of nutrition for long. Enteral products taken orally can be quite expensive and they aren't very palatable. Tube-based feedings are more practical, and they can be a vital tool in IBD treatment.

Total parenteral nutrition is used when the GI tract isn't accessible or when oral or tube-based feedings have failed. When your gut isn't working well, feeding via a central access device placed into the largest vein of the body becomes your only way to get nutrition. This may be necessary if you have a prolonged bowel obstruction or a fistula with output too high to control with medication or when enteral nutrition doesn't work.

Few studies have been done on total parenteral nutrition as a treatment for IBD, but those that exist suggest that it's less desirable than enteral nutrition. The reason, according to experts in the field, is that total parenteral nutrition doesn't stimulate the gut or provide a fuel source for the microbiome, meaning that it's not helpful for maintaining the integrity of the gut. People who receive total parenteral nutrition are at risk of central line infections, which can be life-threatening. Despite the downsides, for some people with IBD, this is the only way to get proper nutrition. If you're unable to take in adequate calories by mouth or enteral means, total parenteral nutrition may become part of your overall treatment plan.

DIETS SPECIFICALLY FOR IBD

You may have considered trying a specific diet for treating IBD promoted in the media or in other books. Doctors and dietitians are asked all the time about the best diet out there.

One of the more popular diets is the Specific Carbohydrate Diet, as described in the book *Breaking the Vicious Cycle* by Elaine Gottschall. It's based on the theory that carbohydrates are the primary source of intestinal bacteria that contribute to IBD. Dr. Gottschall claims that the diet, which consists of a grain-, lactose- and sucrose-free regimen, cured her daughter's colitis. The diet prohibits:
• All grains, including corn, oats and rice.
• Sugar, sucrose, fructose and high-fructose corn syrup.

- Canned vegetables.
- Canned/processed meats.
- Starchy tubers (potatoes, yams, parsnips).
- Bread, pasta and other starchy foods.
- Milk, most milk products and ice cream.
- Candy, chocolate, margarine and ketchup.

So, what's left to eat, you ask?
- Fresh meat, poultry, fish, shellfish and eggs.
- Fresh or frozen vegetables.
- Legumes (beans, lentils, peas).
- Most hard cheeses.
- Honey.
- Most fruits and nuts.
- Coffee, tea and juices with no additives.

There have been no scientifically controlled studies on a large enough scale to suggest that this diet works in treating IBD. No studies prove it to be a cure. However, several small-scale studies, particularly in children, indicate that the diet has some promising benefits in IBD remission.

The diet isn't inherently harmful, but it's certainly not one that most people would be able to follow for a long time. Almost all of the foods in the diet have to be prepared at home using flour made from almonds or other nuts and honey as the sugar source. In her book, Dr. Gottschall says that the diet will not be successful unless you strictly adhere to it, with no deviations. Following such rigid rules could place you at risk of malnutrition if you end up over-restricting your intake.

With these caveats in mind, there's no reason you can't follow this diet if you feel that it gives you some control over the state of your health and that you can meet your nutritional needs while following it. Understand that there are no guarantees about how it will work for you.

Other popular books on gut-related diets include books that focus on a restrictive diet, on spiritual healing or a combination of the two, as well as a series of books on eating for your blood type. The blood type series covers a variety of different conditions, not just IBD, which is one reason to be wary of the claims. How can a single type of diet help Crohn's disease, irritable bowel syndrome, peptic ulcer and diverticulitis? No large-scale studies have looked at any of these approaches or indicated a therapeutic benefit.

Another diet that's recently begun to garner some attention with regard to IBD is the Mediterranean diet. This diet became popular in the United States after multiyear studies found people who reside along the Mediterranean Sea have far lower rates of death from cardiovascular disease and cancer, as well as lower incidences of Alzheimer's dementia and type 2 diabetes. Hallmarks of the Mediterranean diet are its high content of olive oil, fruits, vegetables and nuts, along with limited to moderate amounts of animal-based proteins.

With regard to IBD, a couple of recent studies have compared a Mediterranean-style diet to the Specific Carbohydrate Diet. As in previous studies, nearly 50% of both groups experienced remission of symptoms. Given these data, the increased overall intake of vegetables and fruits with these diets is likely what's beneficial for individuals with IBD. Vegetables and fruits stimulate the microbiome, repairing the gut and maintaining a healthy integrity.

While the Specific Carbohydrate Diet has been shown to be relatively equal to the Mediterranean diet in its ability to maintain remission in people with Crohn's disease, the Mediterranean diet seems to be a much more pragmatic option because it doesn't involve any rigid, hard-to-follow rules.

To date, no one particular diet has been shown to change the overall course of IBD in significant numbers of people. You may read or hear of many different miracle diets. Remind yourself that if one of these diets was truly a miracle cure, it would receive widespread attention and adoption. Changing your diet to gain more control over symptoms and to improve your health is a positive step, but altering your diet won't cure your disease.

Eating during a flare

The following menus are for specific situations that a person with IBD may encounter. They are based on what we understand about IBD flares, the characteristics of specific foods and the need to avoid malnutrition. We encourage you to use these menus as a starting place to help determine which foods can help you best manage your IBD. In other words, they're suggestions, not rigid rules.

This sample eating plan provides about 7 grams of fiber, nearly all soluble, over the course of a day.

Breakfast:
- ½ cup regular Cream of Wheat cereal. Stir in ½ teaspoon smooth peanut butter, ½ teaspoon sugar or honey, and cinnamon to taste. Top with ¼ cup lactose-free milk (or regular cow's milk if it doesn't bother you).
- 2 scrambled eggs
- 1 small, ripe banana

Midmorning snack:
- 1 cup lactose-free nutrition supplement or 1 cup yogurt without fruit
- 6 saltine crackers
- ½ teaspoon smooth peanut butter

Lunch:
- 1 cup chicken noodle soup combined with ¼ cup finely chopped canned carrots
- ½ slice white bread, lightly toasted, topped with sliced hard-boiled egg and light mayonnaise
- 3 to 4 slices canned peaches (not halves, because they may still have the skin intact, whereas slices tend to be peeled)

Afternoon snack:
- 3 saltines topped with canned tuna, mixed with small amount of mayonnaise or substitute. It's OK to use a small amount of onion powder for flavoring, if it doesn't bother you.
- 1 cup lactose-free nutrition supplement

Dinner:
- 3 to 4 ounces broiled salmon
- ½ cup boiled, peeled zucchini (no need

to seed) with small amount of salt, pepper or both
- Small boiled or mashed potato with skin removed, with ½ teaspoon butter and small amount of salt and/or pepper
- ½ cup applesauce

Evening snack:
- 2 white-flour crackers, each topped with 1 teaspoon smooth peanut butter
- 1 cup lactose-free nutrition supplement or yogurt without fruit

Substitutions:
If you get tired of these foods, start to make substitutions, but do so without adding additional fiber or lactose (unless lactose-containing dairy products don't bother you when you aren't in a flare).

Be aware that sometimes you'll be able to eat these foods with no problems, but other times they may make your other symptoms worse. It's helpful to keep track of what you're eating and how you're reacting to the foods in a food diary so you can spot trends and stick with what works.
- Instead of Cream of Wheat, try Cream of Rice or a packet of plain instant oatmeal with no added flavorings or fruit pieces. If you want to get back to dry cereal, try Rice Krispies.
- Instead of chicken noodle soup, try any broth: meat, poultry, fish or vegetable. Bone broth has more protein than standard broth. Substitute white rice or small pieces of boiled, skinless potato for the noodles. For added protein, stir a beaten egg into the hot broth with a fork, or add very tender pieces of lean, skinless cooked meat.

- For lactose-free nutrition supplements, try whey isolate-based products that are unflavored and can be added to items like broth, soup or mashed potatoes.
- For fruit, try canned varieties of peaches, apricots, or pineapple in small amounts. Start with a few small pieces one day and wait a day or two as you find your tolerance level before adding any more. Fresh cantaloupe, watermelon and honeydew melons have little fiber and they're mostly soluble and tolerated well.
- Instead of mayonnaise, use any salad dressing you like, as long as it doesn't contain pieces of vegetable or herb particles. You can strain those bits out of a favorite bottled dressing with a coffee filter before using it. You can flavor your own oil and vinegar with your choice of herbs, but strain it before using it.
- Instead of saltines or soda crackers, use any type of cracker made of plain white flour with no added fiber, bran, whole grains or seeds. Oyster crackers or water crackers are examples.
- Instead of canned tuna, try canned salmon, any fish without bones or smoked oysters. You'll probably do better without the stringier shellfish, such as fresh, smoked or canned clams or shrimp.
- Instead of broiled salmon, try a fresh or frozen fish fillet such as tilapia, cod, halibut or whitefish without skin or bones. Breading may have preservatives or extra sodium in it, so try it without breading. Broil or steam until very soft. Canned fish is also acceptable.
- For vegetables, try canned, including green beans, skinless and seedless

tomatoes, tomato sauce or paste, mushrooms or asparagus. Small amounts of finely chopped cucumber without skin or seeds are OK.

- Instead of peanut butter, try any nut butter that's been very finely ground and contains no chunks, but use small quantities (1 to 2 teaspoons at a time). Cashew or almond butter is often available in grocery stores.

When you start to feel better

As your symptoms begin to subside, you can start reintroducing a small amount of fiber into your diet, along with a few of your favorite foods, as long as you can tolerate them. The smartest way to do this is to change one meal or snack at a time and add the food in small amounts.

Begin with a breakfast, lunch or dinner. On day one, eat a half portion. If you experience no adverse side effects by the next day, eat a half portion again on days two and three. On the morning of day four, if you're still feeling well, you can start eating the full amount. If you're still doing fine after a week, substitute another meal or snack for one you've been eating during your flare. If you encounter problems, go back a step until you feel better. Then, try again, but instead of changing an entire meal or a snack at a time, change only one food.

Writing down what changes you make and how you feel after you eat something new can be helpful. If you connect a particular food with unpleasant symptoms, eliminate that food for a while until

you feel better. If that particular food is one of your favorites, try it again, starting with a very small amount. You may be able to tolerate a little of it once every four or five days. Even though that may not be as often as you like, it's better than not being able to eat it at all.

The sample menu that follows has a few more grams of fiber and a few more calories. But it's best to continue to eat small, frequent meals rather than eating too much at one time.

Breakfast:

- ¾ cup Special K cereal with ⅓ cup lactose-free milk (or regular cow's milk if it doesn't bother you) and ½ teaspoon sugar, if desired.
- 1 peeled, ripe plum. Peeling is important. Most skins contain insoluble fiber, which may be too advanced at this stage. The pulp contains soluble fiber, which should help you gain confidence in increasing your variety of foods. Even though some skins contain pectin, a soluble fiber, they're tough and may be abrasive, so it's best to avoid them.

Midmorning snack:

- ½ slice white toast with 1 teaspoon smooth peanut butter and a little seedless jelly

Lunch:

- ½ cup pureed vegetable soup. Dilute a canned variety with water as directed and blend until smooth.
- Tuna salad on ½ piece white toast. Mix tuna with light mayonnaise and a little onion powder and small amount of dill.
- 1 cup watermelon chunks

Afternoon snack:
- ½ skinless, boneless chicken breast, boiled and dipped in a blend of soy sauce and either fresh ground or powdered ginger

Dinner:
- 3 to 4 ounces shredded chicken or turkey breast
- ½ cup mashed potatoes with small amount of turkey gravy
- ½ cup canned green beans
- Small piece of spice cake topped with small amount of powdered sugar

Evening snack:
- ½ cup applesauce with a bit of cinnamon, if desired
- ½ toasted white English muffin with 1 teaspoon margarine or peanut butter

Substitutions:
- For juice, try any kind of fruit juice without pulp.
- For fruit, try any fresh or canned fruit without noticeably tough skins or seeds.
- For bread, try any white bread or cracker — no whole grains.
- For cereals, try any kind with less than 2 grams of fiber and less than 6 grams of sugar in one cup. Examples are Rice Krispies, corn flakes, Crispix, Special K and Corn Chex. There are others, so read the labels.
- For vegetables, try any kind of canned vegetables without hard seeds or tough skins. Avoid corn and legumes, such as peas, kidney beans, navy beans, pinto beans, lentils or chili beans.
- Instead of turkey, chicken or fish, try any tender, moist meat that doesn't

have gristle or tough connective tissue.
- Instead of spice cake, try a soft cookie made with white flour or ginger snaps dipped in tea or milk.

Getting back to normal

If you've tolerated the addition of small amounts of fiber and sugar and larger portions without ill effects, you can begin to normalize your diet even more.

Breakfast:
- ¾ cup cooked instant oatmeal with 1 teaspoon honey and ½ cup lactose-free milk (or regular cow's milk if it doesn't bother you)
- 2 scrambled eggs
- 1 cup berries

Midmorning snack:
- ½ banana
- ½ graham cracker with 1 teaspoon smooth peanut or almond butter
- 2 string cheese

Lunch:
- 1 cup egg-drop soup with oyster crackers. Stir a beaten egg into boiling chicken broth
- Tuna sandwich on white or wheat bread. Mix 3 ounces tuna with mayonnaise or salad dressing and 1 large, chopped lettuce leaf
- ½ peeled apple or 6 mandarin orange sections

Afternoon snack:
- A few ounces of pickled herring or smoked salmon on saltine crackers
- 4 to 5 grapes (peeled the first time)

Dinner:
- 3 to 4 ounces of pressure-cooked or very tender chicken
- ½ cup mashed potatoes or white rice with a little margarine or gravy
- ½ cup very soft cooked broccoli or carrots
- ¼ ripe medium cantaloupe

When you've recovered from a flare

If you're still tolerating newer foods and larger portions well, you can move on to the next step. Try the following foods by adding them to your diet in small doses, one at a time. These foods have more protein and quite a bit more fiber than the previous ones to ensure that you receive adequate nutrients.

If you're trying a food for the first time, experiment with it peeled and cooked first, over the course of several days, before eating it with the skin or raw.

Breakfast (2 options):
- Egg omelet with small amounts of well-cooked onion, garlic, tomato (seeds and skin removed, if trying for the first time), peeled zucchini or other summer squash, and/or chopped cooked spinach, kale or chard
- 1 slice wheat toast with margarine and jelly, if desired
- ½ cup frozen hash browns cooked in small amount of olive or canola oil
- 1 cup berries

or
- 1 cup instant or quick oatmeal with 1 teaspoon smooth peanut butter, ½ sliced banana, and ¼ to ½ cup skim cow's milk or lactose-free milk
- 1 cup berries
- 1 teaspoon ground flaxseeds

Lunch:
- 1 cup canned tomato/vegetable-based soup or meat-based soup with ½ cup (per 2 cups liquid) added canned vegetables of your choice (no corn or cooked dried beans)
- Chicken or turkey sandwich with 1 to 2 slices wheat or rye toast, mayonnaise or salad dressing, 1 lettuce leaf, and 1 slice tomato
- 4 to 6 sweet potato chips
- ½ orange

Dinner:
- ½ marinated baked chicken breast
- ½ cup mashed winter squash
- ½ cup white rice
- ½ cup well-cooked or canned asparagus
- 8 ounces low-fat milk

Snacks:
- Smooth nut butter on white flour crackers (crackers with whole grains or seeds can be incorporated in small amounts over time)
- Applesauce
- Peeled, seedless fruit (before advancing to whole fruit)
- Fruit juice, either clear or with small amounts of pulp
- V8 or tomato juice
- Low-fat yogurt
- Pickled herring, sardines, smoked oysters, smoked clams, fish pâté on crackers made from white flour
- Gelatin desserts
- Pudding

GENERAL GUIDELINES FOR HEALTHY EATING

Variety is important when it comes to a healthy diet. Taking even one bite of 20 to 30 different plant-based foods each week can make a notable impact on your ability to stave off flares. That's because a wide range of healthy foods helps ensure that your gut microbiome is composed of diverse bacteria.

If you struggle to consume enough food, or if you're taking certain medications to treat your IBD, or both, it's very important to get adequate vitamins and minerals. If you reach the point that you need help with your diet, talk to your health care provider. Nutritional guidance can be overwhelming, and it's best to try not to overcomplicate things.

At the end of the day, the most important thing is that you're nourished and you're tolerating your food as best you can. Keep things simple and balanced, and do what you can to eat well.

Here are some additional suggestions for eating healthily:

IBD NUTRITION TERMS

Enteral nutrition. Nutrition provided directly to the gastrointestinal tract through a feeding tube. It can be placed through the nose for short-term use or through the skin directly into the stomach or intestines for long-term use.

Enzymes. Proteins that help speed up chemical reactions in the body related to the building up or breaking down of substances.

Gluten. A protein consisting of gliadin and glutenin found in wheat, barley and rye.

Lactase enzyme. An enzyme produced in the body that breaks down lactose, a sugar found in milk and milk products.

Lactose. The primary natural sugar in milk.

Low-fiber diet. A diet that contains less than 13 grams of fiber per day. Some health care providers or facilities define it differently.

Low-residue diet. A diet low in fiber or certain other foods, which often results in retained contents in the large intestine.

Macronutrients. The nutrients your body uses in the largest amounts — carbohydrates, protein and fats.

- *Get plenty of omega-3s.* Use mostly olive oil for salads and olive oil and canola oil for cooking. Eat fish often. Omega-3 fatty acids found in these oils and fish and other seafood help reduce inflammation. It's possible to get omega-3 fatty acids from plant sources, such as walnut and flaxseed oils, but that means your body has to perform a chemical conversion that isn't very effective. Fish such as herring, salmon, halibut, flounder and swordfish are highest in omega-3s. However, you may need to reduce fish consumption if you're pregnant because of the poten-tial for mercury in fish. Avoid large amounts of soy, safflower, corn, cotton-seed, sunflower and peanut oils. They contain omega-6 fatty acids, which promote inflammation.
- *Eat small, frequent meals.* You want to avoid getting too full or asking your digestive tract to process a lot of food at once. At the same time, you need additional calories and protein to repair damaged tissue. By eating small amounts frequently, you're better able to meet those requirements without distending your gut and causing bloat-ing, cramps and changes in bowel habits.

Malnutrition. An acute, subacute or chronic state of nutrition in which varying degrees of undernutrition or overnutrition produce changes in body composition and cause diminished function.

Metabolism. Chemical reactions in living cells necessary to convert food into usable energy, supplying the body the energy it needs to function.

Micronutrients. Required nutrients present in the body in minute quantities — vitamins, trace elements and minerals.

Oral nutritional supplement. Supplemental protein or a meal replacement avail-able in powder, ready-to-drink, bar or cookie forms.

Parenteral nutrition. Intravenous administration of nutrition (protein, carbohy-drate, fat, minerals, electrolytes, vitamins and other trace elements) to individuals who can't eat them or absorb them by other methods.

Residue. Fiber, undigested food, bacteria, intestinal secretions and intestinal cells that have sloughed off, found in the gastrointestinal tract.

Short-chain fatty acids. The fatty acids acetate, propionate and butyrate that arise from the fermentation of fibers in the colonic microbiota.

- *Avoid foods and beverages high in fat and sugar.* They attract a lot of water to the colon, which can irritate your gastrointestinal tract. The result may be bloating, a feeling of fullness, cramping and rapid emptying of your bowels.
- *Drink a lot of fluids.* Water is generally best. It helps move fiber through your bowels.
- *Use a pressure cooker.* It makes meat and vegetables very tender and breaks down their fibers so they're easier for your gut to tolerate. Think of it as starting the digestive process during cooking.

Navigating nutrition advice for IBD is quite the journey. At times, it can be frustrating, and food may seem like the enemy. However, eating is essential to life, so food choice can be a vital tool for managing your disease. Changing what you eat can help your recovery and reduce flares, but a healthy diet isn't a cure. It's just one component of a comprehensive treatment plan. The important thing is to eat a variety of healthy foods to stay as well nourished as possible.

11

Taking charge of your lifestyle

A variety of events and circumstances in your life can affect your ability to cope with IBD. Not all of them are under your control. It's important to manage those that you do have control over.

PAIN

Abdominal pain can be a constant problem for some people with IBD. The pain can come from many different sources. Sometimes, pain can be very difficult to manage. You may feel uncomfortable discussing your pain with your doctors. It's easy to feel judged, especially if your laboratory results are typical and you aren't "supposed" to be in pain.

Pain is hard to deal with emotionally — not just physically. People in pain feel vulnerable and at the mercy of those treating them. The key is to have a strong partnership with your health care provider so you can work together to problem-solve your issues.

One of the reasons pain is difficult to manage is that doctors don't have a good way of objectively measuring it. What's very painful to one person is only slightly bothersome to someone else. We all have different pain thresholds. You may feel frustrated because your predominant symptom is pain, and your health care provider is telling you that nothing is wrong. What that means is that he or she can't find anything abnormal on tests. It doesn't mean you don't have pain.

What can help is to keep an accurate diary of your pain and to be as specific as you can about what you're experiencing and when. For example, do you feel pain all of the time or intermittently? Is the pain more of a dull ache or sharp and stabbing? Is it worse after meals or at night? What makes it better? Is it always in the same place or does it move?

Some common reasons for pain include active disease, an obstruction in the intestines, irritability of the gastrointestinal tract and side effects from medication. Pain in your gut could also be coming from something totally unrelated to your IBD. Remember, having IBD doesn't make you immune to other conditions.

Withdrawal from narcotics can also cause rebound pain. Unfortunately, it's possible to become addicted to narcotics if you take them for a long time and your body gets used to the medication. You may experience worse pain when you stop the narcotics.

Sometimes, even after a thorough work-up — including blood and stool tests, X-rays and maybe even a colonoscopy — there's no obvious explanation for the pain. One possibility is what's called neuropathic pain, which is pain that originates from irritated nerve fibers along the wall of the bowel or inside the abdominal wall itself. This is also known as visceral hypersensitivity. It's a condition in which the nerves are overly sensitive, signaling pain in situations that typically don't produce pain.

This type of pain can be more difficult to treat than other types, so it takes a multipronged approach to manage it. A nonnarcotic approach is a type of medication called a tricyclic antidepressant, which reduces discomfort by blocking pain signals from the gut to the brain. Keep in mind that it may not be possible to completely eliminate pain. The goal is to keep it at a minimum so that it doesn't interfere with day-to-day functioning.

Doctors generally only perform surgery to help manage a person's pain in the case of very active disease, an obstruction or an obvious mechanical abnormality that's painful.

STRESS

Stress falls into that odd category of being hard to define, but you know it when you feel it. Stress can be positive, such as stress that may accompany a new job, a wedding or a new life adventure. Stress can also be negative, such as stress that accompanies being stuck in a traffic jam, being overwhelmed at work or dealing with death or divorce.

Simply defined, stress is a deviation from the norm that you're powerless to avoid. It can be brief, such as worrying about missing a day of work due to illness. Or it can be chronic, such as juggling the ongoing demands of work, caring for your kids and caring for your parents. We all know that stress is bad for us and can take a toll on our bodies in different ways. Although stress doesn't cause IBD, it can certainly make it worse or even unmask the disease in someone who hasn't yet been diagnosed.

Interestingly, there seems to be a connection between IBD, stress and the immune system. Researchers are just beginning to understand the relationship between the human immune system and the body's stress response. Because everyone is different, it's difficult to scientifically test for the mechanisms by which stress affects the immune system and its function. That's partly because everyone deals with stress differently, and what's stressful to one person isn't so for someone else.

It's important to recognize your own personal stress triggers — what causes you stress — and deal with them. Don't expect that you can ever totally avoid stress; it's not possible. But making purposeful choices to avoid or limit excessive stress is always a good strategy.

Take the end-of-the-year holiday season, for example. Talk about stress! Even though holidays are supposed to be joyous, studies show that more people become depressed and stressed around the holidays than any other time of the year. There are many obstacles to enjoying yourself. Plus, for people with IBD, there's extra temptation with seasonal foods and holiday gatherings. This can be hard on your digestive system.

It probably doesn't surprise you to know that doctors tend to get the most calls from patients in distress around the holidays. Consider preparing for this time of year in terms of your schedule and diet as much as you can, and don't stop taking your medication. There's no holiday from your disease and the need to keep inflammation at bay. Preventive steps will help you avoid a flare.

One other note: There's a misperception among doctors and the public that people who are high-strung or have type A personalities are more at risk of IBD. This isn't true. People of all personality types, ethnicities and cultures get IBD. Healthy, proactive techniques to relieve stress can be a means to control disease symptoms that seem to be driven by stress.

ANXIETY AND DEPRESSION

Many people with IBD experience anxiety or depression, or both, as part of their illness. It's important to understand this is common, and managing anxiety and depression can impact how you feel and your ability to cope with your symptoms. This doesn't imply that you're causing your symptoms. It means that if you can reduce your anxiety and depression, this can make a difference in how you feel physically. Imagine the following scenarios.

Scenario 1. You have an exciting day planned. You're going on a hike with a close friend. You woke up to find the weather perfect for your outing and you can't wait to get started. As you're walking out the door, you realize that you forgot your water bottle, and you race back to the kitchen and grab it. On your way back to the front door, you're so excited that you don't notice a chair in your path and stub your toe on the chair. Ouch! It hurts, but you're focused on meeting your friend and off you go!

Scenario 2. You're home sitting around, feeling sad and lonely. A friend that you wanted to spend time with has made other plans, and you're feeling a little rejected. You're also stewing about how your boss criticized your work during a meeting a couple of days ago. And you're behind on your rent. On the way to the kitchen for some water, you stub your toe and it hurts — a lot!

It's possible that in scenario 1 you stubbed your toe even harder than in scenario 2. But because of the exciting day you have planned, you notice it less. The positive events of the day outweigh the negatives.

You can't wish away anxiety and depression, but there are strategies that you can use to help manage them and improve how you feel overall. Talk to your health care provider about the benefits of cognitive behavioral therapy and meeting with a good therapist. Working with a psychologist or psychiatrist can be helpful. Cognitive behavioral therapy is a commonly used tool for management of anxiety and depression.

SLEEP AND FATIGUE

It's easy to overlook your need for a good night's sleep and downplay its importance. But good sleep is central to good health. Experts agree that most people should get seven to eight hours of uninterrupted sleep a night. Among people with IBD, however, sleep may be cut short or interrupted by diarrhea, pain or other symptoms. This can start a vicious cycle in which you're constantly ill because you can't get adequate rest. Discuss persistent fatigue or excessive sleepiness with your health care provider. These issues can be a signal of ongoing inflammation or another condition, such as sleep apnea.

Some people take prescription sleeping pills because they have difficulty falling asleep or have trouble staying asleep. Others use narcotics for this purpose. Most sleeping pills won't interact with medicines used to treat IBD, but they can be addictive. It's important to understand why you aren't getting enough sleep. Sleeping pills aren't a cure for the problem. What about melatonin? Melatonin is a hormone that the body produces to help regulate the brain's awake-sleep cycle. Melatonin, available over the counter in stores and pharmacies, might be a safer alternative to prescription pills.

Sometimes, fatigue is the only symptom of active inflammation, so let your health care provider know if you seem more fatigued than normal. If your IBD seems to be under control and you're still really tired, keep pressing the issue. You might want a workup to look for other causes.

Fatigue is one of those highly nonspecific symptoms. It often takes some digging to figure out why someone feels tired all the time. Sure, having active IBD can wear you out, but doctors see patients who are fatigued and aren't having an active bout of inflammation. The fatigue may be occurring for other reasons, such as a medication side effect, depression, high blood sugar (glucose), low iron levels, an underactive thyroid, sleep apnea or simply a lack of sleep.

Anemia, a reduction in healthy red blood cells, is often undertreated in people with IBD. Health care providers may assume that anemia is normal in a person with IBD, given that the disease can cause bleeding and impair a person's ability to absorb iron. If you're feeling fatigued, make sure that you're checked for anemia and receive proper treatment if you have a deficiency.

Once you find the cause of fatigue, it generally can be treated. Fatigue doesn't have to keep you from doing the things you want to and should be doing.

TOBACCO USE

If you have Crohn's disease and you smoke, the most important change that you can make is to stop smoking. Research shows that smoking cigarettes increases both your risk and your family's risk of developing Crohn's disease, and it worsens the progression of the disease. Even secondhand smoke increases the risk of Crohn's disease in the children of smokers. Women are particularly vulnerable. Several studies have shown that women smokers who have Crohn's disease need more steroids, have more surgeries, experience flares earlier and don't respond as well to medications. As few as five cigarettes a day can worsen your disease, as does exposure to secondhand smoke.

There are many ways to successfully quit smoking, some of which you may not have heard about, so ask your health care provider about your options. This is a very important step in managing Crohn's disease.

Strangely, ulcerative colitis occurs less often in people who smoke. It's when they quit that they tend to develop the disease or experience a flare. Still, smoking doesn't convey protection against developing colitis, and it has many bad effects, so doctors encourage all individuals with IBD to kick the habit.

PHYSICAL ACTIVITY

Physical activity is important for your overall health. Understandably, when your IBD is active, you may not feel up to exercising. But when your IBD is in remission, we encourage you to take part in regular physical activity. The benefits of exercise include a sense of well-being, stronger bones and weight control, to name a few.

For most people with IBD, the only restrictions to activity are what you impose on yourself. Physical activity tends to rev up the bowel, as you may have already noticed. Some people feel nervous when they're exercising and don't know the location of a nearby bathroom. Others train for and run marathons or participate in long, group bike rides. If having a bathroom close by is your concern, instead of going for a walk, exercise at a gym or fitness club or in your own home.

Find a few activities that you enjoy, and work on your strength and endurance. If you don't think you have time for exercise or if you have trouble making yourself do it, consider getting a dog. A dog demands that you get some exercise, even if it's only taking the dog for a walk around the block. A dog also can be an excellent companion when you're not feeling well. Pets tend to be stress reducers.

TRAVEL

Having IBD doesn't mean that you can't travel. It's important to get away and see the world. Here are some travel tips for comfortable and safe travel.

- Always make sure you have enough medication with you when you're away from home, even if you're only going to work.
- Check your intravenous (IV) medication schedule before making travel plans.
- If possible, choose travel that allows you to control your food and water supply and that provides adequate access to a bathroom.
- When planning international travel, be sure to understand vaccination recommendations and requirements as well as any epidemic alerts that have been issued. Because management of IBD may include use of steroids, immuno-suppressants or biologics, vaccines made from live viruses (which you have no way to fight off) can harm you. These include vaccines against polio, yellow fever, chickenpox and rotavirus.
- Discuss your travel plans in advance with your health care provider. He or she may recommend nonprescription therapies for traveler's diarrhea or prescribe antibiotics to take with you. If you're traveling to a place that requires proof of vaccination and you haven't been vaccinated because of the medications you're taking, a letter from your doctor stating this is required.
- Consider packing your own toilet paper or wipes in your carry-on luggage.
- Have an emergency travel kit that includes a change of underwear, disposable underpants or liners, a roll of your favorite toilet paper, toilet wipes or a cream (like Balneol) that can be used on toilet paper.

Ally's Law, first passed in the Illinois senate, was championed by a little girl from Chicago who was turned away from the employee bathrooms at a clothing store when she had an urgent need to have a bowel movement. She had an embarrassing accident and was infuriated. The law grants people with medical needs access to bathroom facilities at stores and other places that don't otherwise offer public services. You can get a free card to carry in your wallet by contacting your local Crohn's & Colitis Foundation chapter or printing one from the Inflammatory Bowel Disease Center website (see page 183).

WORK

Having IBD means there's a good chance you'll miss some time at work because of disease flares and doctor appointments. There are laws in place to prevent chronic illness-based discrimination in the workplace. In general, employers must make accommodations for an employee with a physical disability who is otherwise competent to fulfill a position.

Before accepting a job, understand what's expected of you and how the job may be modified, if necessary, to fit your needs.

Only you can decide if and when to tell your boss or colleagues about your ulcerative colitis or Crohn's disease. If your work environment is supportive, you may be able to tell people about the struggles you endure and the accommodations you need. However, the world isn't always sympathetic to people with illnesses, and it's important to use common sense about when, how and to whom you disclose information about your condition. An attorney can advise you how and when to inform your employer or potential employer about your IBD.

With regard to your employer, try to predict how accommodating and compassionate he or she may be based on his or her interactions with other colleagues who've faced health challenges. Most employers generally want their employees to be happy because it maximizes productivity. If you need someone to lean on at work, colleagues can sometimes be a better choice than your boss. They may be more understanding. But, again, use caution. Some colleagues may be supportive, and others may gossip or believe that you're getting special treatment because of your medical condition.

Remember that most people have no idea what having IBD means, so what you say and how you say it will make all the difference. If you choose to tell people, be honest and clear about your illness and your needs and do so in a calm way. If you're emotional, people are more likely to be concerned that your work may be negatively impacted by your IBD, or vice versa. If you present your illness as a challenge that you're able to rise up to, while still needing some accommodations, people will be less likely to see it as a barrier to your productivity and will be more likely to help out.

So, what's the bottom line? If you trust the people you work for and with, it may be productive to tell them about your IBD and ask for the help and accommodations you need.

At work:
- Be clear about the accommodations you need, such as a work location that's close to the bathroom.
- When considering job opportunities, keep your disease in mind and choose a job that has some schedule flexibility.
- During flares, request assignments that don't require long periods of time away from bathroom facilities.
- Today, many jobs can be performed from home. Ask if you can work remotely, either permanently or during flares.

Sometimes it may be appropriate to take short-term disability leave from work to get your health on track. Short-term disability periods tend to last about three months. Permanent disability is an option if your disease symptoms are so unpredictable that trying to hold down even a part-time job is difficult. The Crohn's & Colitis Foundation is an excellent resource for help with determining whether permanent disability is right for you (see page 183).

Sex, fertility and pregnancy

12

Talking about sex with anyone may feel awkward, and it can be more difficult if the other person is someone you think may not understand or be sympathetic to your situation. Fortunately, however, many people are comfortable asking questions about engaging in sexual intercourse. For almost everyone with IBD, having sex doesn't cause stress that would lead to an IBD flare. Having sexual intercourse may actually make you feel more normal, because for many people, sex plays an important role in creating a sense of well-being.

On the other hand, engaging in physical intimacy may bring up fears about incontinence or needing a bathroom at an inopportune time. You may be self-conscious about changes in your appearance due to the disease or the cosmetic side effects from steroids, surgery or an ostomy. Because of your disease, body parts and areas that were meant to be involved in intimacy likely have been poked and prodded by people other than intimate partners.

Many people with IBD will say, "I've been through so much; I have no privacy left." It may be that certain body parts are now associated with negative feelings versus warm, positive ones. If that's the case for you, communicate this to your sexual partners so they understand if you're resistant to certain sexual practices and so their feelings don't get hurt when you aren't in the mood.

There are specially trained psychologists who can help with counseling and reaffirmation of your sexuality. Ask your health care provider to refer you to one, if possible. Support groups may also provide a way to gather information about sensitive issues (see Chapter 11). Please don't stay silent; if you don't talk about your issues and concerns, they won't get resolved.

MEN

Men with IBD tend to be most concerned about whether they can perform sexually. It's reassuring to them that the disease doesn't appear to increase the risk of erectile dysfunction. Active inflammation from IBD rarely causes erectile problems, but one of the causes of erectile dysfunction is undiagnosed or untreated depression. Watch for signs of depression in yourself and get the help you need.

Loss of libido can result from physical discomfort and symptoms of active IBD. It also may be associated with a decreased testosterone level. Testosterone is a sex hormone made from cholesterol. If your body lacks adequate levels of cholesterol because of diarrhea or poor absorption in your intestines, your body can't produce enough testosterone. Among men with IBD found to have low testosterone, improving nutrition and wearing a testosterone patch are ways to increase testosterone.

One of the risks of having a J pouch is that you may have retrograde ejaculation after the surgery. In this condition, during orgasm, semen enters the bladder instead of emerging through the penis. Fortunately, this complication is becoming less common as surgeons gain more experience with J-pouch surgery.

Men with IBD are also concerned about their ability to father children and the likelihood of passing the disease to the next generation. Preliminary genetic studies have suggested that the risk of passing along IBD is stronger from the mother than from the father, but that hasn't been proven conclusively. Overall, there's no difference in sperm health in men with and without IBD. There's no convincing data to suggest that medications used to treat IBD such as methotrexate, thiopurines or biologics affect sperm quality. An exception is sulfasalazine, which significantly lowers sperm count. However, this is reversed when you stop taking the drug. The sperm-lowering effect isn't dose dependent, which means it would happen even if you took only one tablet a day.

WOMEN

IBD symptoms are consistently rated as more severe by women than by men. Both men and women are concerned with attractiveness, intimacy and sexual performance. Women, however, tend to have greater concerns about self-image, and they're more fearful about having children.

Active disease can lead to fatigue and loss of libido, in addition to the embarrassment of fecal incontinence — more good reasons to try to keep your disease in remission. Of all the medications used, steroids are the most problematic.

Stacey had fairly well-controlled ulcerative colitis, but she noticed that the time around her periods definitely included more abdominal cramps and looser stools than the rest of the month. She wasn't sure if these were flares of her IBD. She finally asked if it was normal to have more stools before her period — almost like a "mini flare" every month. Stacey was asked to track her symptoms through two full menstrual cycles. This revealed that during the week before Stacey's period, she had more gastrointestinal symptoms, which went away the following week. Instead of taking steroids to help manage the symptoms, as Stacey had in the past, doctors recommended she be mindful of this relationship and take medications other than steroids to help with abdominal cramps and gastrointestinal symptoms.

They're linked to weight gain, acne and mood swings, all of which contribute to poor self-image.

Crohn's disease that involves the rectum and vagina can be physically deforming, making intercourse painful. If you have an ostomy or other surgical scar, this may also affect your self-esteem. It's difficult to feel sexy or to enjoy sex if you aren't comfortable with who you are and how your body looks and functions.

So, what can you do? Women with Crohn's disease are often told to avoid thong underwear and bikinis because the band can be particularly irritating to the perianal area and irritate skin tags, fissures or fistulas. Women with a stoma often have self-image issues and serious concerns about attracting a partner. Something that can make women feel more comfortable during intimacy is crotchless underwear and teddies, or teddies with snap crotches. These cover the abdominal wall while exposing the groin area, a change-up that sexual partners may find appealing.

Menstruation

Girls diagnosed with IBD before or during puberty may experience a delay in when they get their first period (called menarche). The delay may be caused by chronic inflammation or poor nutrition, which affects the body's ability to produce the necessary sex hormones. Chronic inflammation can shut down normal hormonal signals that the body uses to talk to itself. This can lead to decreased levels of hormones, which can result in irregular or absent periods. Menarche usually occurs once active disease is treated appropriately.

Disease activity can affect the menstrual cycle and produce irregular or skipped periods or an increase in symptoms before or during the time of menstruation. Studies suggest that women with IBD have more gastrointestinal-related symptoms during their periods than do women in the general population. Gastrointestinal symptoms generally occur in a predictable fashion at the same time every month and include diarrhea, abdominal pain and constipation.

Many women experience worse IBD symptoms either right before or during their periods, sometimes referred to as "mini flares." These symptoms are often related to hormonal changes in the function of the intestines rather than increased inflammation. Be conservative in treating the symptoms, because they tend to go away a few days after your period.

Be careful of over-the-counter medications for menstrual symptoms, which may contain high doses of naproxen sodium or aspirin. These products can cause additional inflammation (see Chapter 6) and damage the lining of the gastrointestinal tract. Your doctor may advise you not to use these medications unless absolutely necessary because of the risk of a disease flare.

Some women have such debilitating gastrointestinal symptoms related to menstruation that stopping their periods altogether is the only way to provide relief. This can be achieved with short-term injectable contraceptives (Depo-Provera) or hormones (Lupron). IBD symptoms aren't a reason to have a hysterectomy, but women who've had surgery for gynecologic problems or other reasons for which a hysterectomy was necessary find that their intestinal symptoms often improve.

Menopause

Women with ulcerative colitis are no more likely to enter menopause early than those without IBD. However, some data suggest that women with Crohn's disease may go through menopause earlier than women without IBD. Researchers have yet to discover why this is.

Menopause leads to many changes in a woman's body. And just as oral contraceptives and pregnancy can help control symptoms of IBD, some gastrointestinal symptoms associated with IBD may decrease in menopause.

That said, a study at Mayo Clinic revealed that postmenopausal women with IBD are just as likely to experience a flare as women who are premenopausal. The study also demonstrated that hormone replacement therapy had a protective effect on IBD disease activity and that this effect appears to be dose dependent. In other words, the higher the hormone replacement therapy dose, the less likely a woman may be to experience a flare. More research needs to be done, however, before hormone replacement therapy can be recommended for women with IBD who are approaching menopause.

Pap tests

Women with IBD who take immunosuppressant drugs, such as steroids and azathioprine or 6-MP, for a long time have an increased risk of cervical abnormalities. An abnormality found during a Pap test can progress and become serious. This is probably related to a reduced ability to clear human papillomavirus (HPV) infection, a common cause of cervical cancer.

Women with IBD who take immunomodulators and certain biologics are also considered at increased risk of HPV and need annual Pap tests with timely follow-up on any abnormal results.

Girls and young women with IBD should be vaccinated for HPV, which is recommended between ages 9 and 26. Recently, the Food and Drug Administration (FDA) approved the HPV vaccine for use in adults ages 27 to 45. The decision to receive the vaccine is made on a case-by-case basis depending on the individual's risk factors for acquiring HPV.

Contraception

Contraception for women with IBD who don't wish to become pregnant differs only slightly from that for women who don't have IBD. The most important goal remains selecting a reliable method of birth control.

Barrier methods such as a condom or diaphragm are acceptable but not quite as effective as other choices, such as birth control pills. Intrauterine devices (IUDs) can be used and are an effective method of contraception. They are often recommended to females with IBD.

Oral contraceptives, or birth control pills, present some challenges for women with IBD. Many antibiotics carry a warning about decreased effectiveness of oral contraceptives when the two are taken in combination; however, not all experts in the field believe this to be true. It may be a theoretical outcome based on what happens in a test tube.

Data regarding the safety of oral contraceptives among women with IBD are conflicting. Some preliminary studies suggest that taking oral contraceptives increases the risk of developing Crohn's disease and ulcerative colitis, but they didn't take into account tobacco use, another risk factor. Reports from Europe, where birth control pills contain a higher amount of estrogen, continue to show modest increases in the risk of developing Crohn's disease, after adjusting for cigarette use. Two U.S. case-control studies, however, found no increased risk of either ulcerative colitis or Crohn's disease from oral contraceptive use.

Other data suggest use of oral contraceptives may worsen IBD. Two small studies in which individuals were followed over a long period of time found that women with Crohn's disease taking oral contraceptives had an increased risk of flares after the disease had gone into remission. No information is available regarding a similar risk in ulcerative colitis.

There are no standard guidelines for oral contraceptive use, in part because there are so many types available (over 70!), so it's an individual decision. Variable amounts of the hormones progesterone and estrogen determine the side effects. In discussions with your health care provider on whether to use an oral contraceptive and which one, consider your overall health, any previous pregnancies and your personal preferences. Select a type that contains the lowest amount of estrogen to lower the risk of blood clots. Because people with IBD also have a tendency to develop blood clots, it's especially risky to take oral contraceptives and smoke — so don't smoke!

FERTILITY AND PREGNANCY

Up to 7% of couples in America are infertile, so don't be too quick to blame your IBD if your efforts to have a baby have been unsuccessful. However, in some circumstances, individuals with IBD do experience decreased fertility.

- Men who take sulfasalazine tend to have a decreased sperm count, but this is totally reversible when stopping the drug.
- Women who have active inflammation may have irregular periods, which decreases the chances of getting pregnant.
- Women with active Crohn's disease may have scarring of their fallopian tubes, making it difficult for an egg to travel from the ovary to the uterus for fertilization.

Females who have a J pouch for colitis are significantly less able to get pregnant than those with ulcerative colitis who haven't had the operation. Construction of the pouch, which sits deep in the pelvis, creates scar tissue thought to prevent eggs from traveling from the ovary to the uterus, so fewer eggs end up in the uterus for possible fertilization. The risk of infertility in someone with a J pouch is about 50% to 60%. Performing the surgery laparoscopically doesn't reduce the risk.

Women with Crohn's disease have slightly lower rates of fertility compared with the general population, probably because of irregular periods and damage to the fallopian tubes.

Females with ulcerative colitis facing surgery who are concerned about future fertility have options. One option is to undergo just the first stage of the surgery and create a temporary stoma until your childbearing is done. The colon is removed but without manipulating the pelvis, which is necessary to remove the rectum and which can cause scarring.

Another option is an operation to attach the small intestine to the rectum. While this protects fertility and doesn't require a stoma, there's still some disease in the rectum. Because the purpose of the surgery is to remove the disease and restore your health, if your rectum has active disease left in place, you may not feel any better after the operation.

Having surgery to create a J pouch, doesn't mean that you'll become infertile, but reduced fertility as a result of scarring is something to keep in mind. Women with J pouches appear to have the standard rate of success using alternative means of becoming pregnant, such as in vitro fertilization.

For women who desire pregnancy and can conceive, having a baby can be exciting, but it can also be quite stressful. Getting pregnant, staying pregnant, delivering and then caring for your newborn can affect your overall health. Most women with IBD are in their childbearing years, and the thought of pregnancy can be quite overwhelming. Be assured that for most women with IBD, pregnancy isn't dangerous. Current medications are leading to better health and longer periods of disease remission.

Planning your pregnancy

Be as proactive as you can about the timing of conception. The healthier you are when conception happens, no matter what your underlying condition may be, the better chance you'll have a successful pregnancy. Discuss with your health care provider the medications you're taking and whether any changes or accommodations need to be made if you get pregnant. For example, if you have reflux disease and take a proton pump inhibitor, this class of medications is considered pretty safe during pregnancy. In fact, because your reflux may worsen during pregnancy, it's important to stay on your medication.

Before you conceive, you may want to meet with a maternal-fetal medicine specialist or your obstetrician to discuss your medications. Pick an obstetrician before you get pregnant, if possible. Inform that individual of your medical history and discuss your medications. Some obstetricians have strong feelings about certain medications, and an open discussion will help avoid problems once you become pregnant. And finally, be aware of gastrointestinal symptoms that commonly occur during pregnancy, such as constipation and reflux, especially during the third trimester.

When you become pregnant, you'll want your health carefully monitored by both a gastroenterologist and your obstetrician for signs of active disease and fetal complications.

How pregnancy affects IBD

If you're in remission at the time of conception, getting pregnant doesn't increase the risk of a flare. The risk of a flare over a nine-month period isn't zero, but being pregnant won't increase it. If, however, you have active disease at the time of conception, the "rule of thirds" comes into play. Approximately one-third

RISK OF IBD IN YOUR CHILD

People with IBD considering pregnancy often want to know what the chances are that they can pass on their disease to a child. As discussed in Chapter 1, the risk of a child getting IBD if only one parent has it is low — between 3% and 7%. If both parents have IBD, then the chance increases to almost 50%. However, it isn't 100%, which indicates that it takes more than genetics alone to develop this disease.

of women will get better, one-third will stay the same and one-third will get worse. Some women say that their disease was never under such good control as when they were pregnant.

A possible reason for the "rule-of-thirds" phenomenon may have to do with the amount of genetic material shared between the mother and the fetus. The more DNA that comes from the father, the more foreign the fetus is to the mother. In order not to reject this foreign entity growing inside her, the mother's body downregulates her own immune system; in the process, her autoimmune disease goes into remission. On the other hand, the more maternal DNA that matches the baby, the worse a woman's disease may be. Again, this applies only to women whose disease is active at the time of conception.

How IBD affects pregnancy

Disease activity at the time of conception is the strongest predictor of pregnancy outcome. Having active IBD during conception is associated with a higher rate of spontaneous abortion. Having active IBD during the course of pregnancy increases the rate of premature births, the chances of the infant being small for its gestational age and the odds of low birth weight. Regardless of disease activity, women with ulcerative colitis or Crohn's disease have higher rates of premature births.

Among women with Crohn's disease, the increased risk of infants having low birth weight and being small for their gestational age may have to do with nutritional factors before and at the time of conception and the fact that more women with Crohn's disease smoke (even during pregnancy) and are more prone to anemia.

Despite some of these sobering statements, most babies born to women with IBD are typical and healthy. Their Apgar scores are in the normal range, and there doesn't appear to be any increased risk for birth defects.

Medications during pregnancy

In general, most medications used to treat IBD are considered low risk during pregnancy. There's some disagreement regarding immunomodulators and biologics, but most experts agree that women with IBD require some type of continued treatment through a pregnancy to keep disease activity under control.

The medications methotrexate, thalidomide and diphenoxylate should be stopped before a planned pregnancy or as soon as pregnancy is determined. Ciprofloxacin shouldn't be taken during pregnancy because of its potential effect on the cartilage of a growing fetus. The drug metronidazole appears to be low risk and can be used for longer periods than previously considered safe.

Mesalamine agents are safe in pregnancy. If you take sulfasalazine, you also need to take folic acid (2 milligrams daily). This is more than what comes in a standard prenatal vitamin. Prednisone is considered low risk during pregnancy if you need it to control IBD; however, there's an increased risk of gestational diabetes and high-birth-weight babies. Cleft palate has been associated with steroid use during pregnancy, but this appears to be linked to asthmatic mothers and not mothers with IBD.

The use of azathioprine and 6-MP has been controversial, but now doctors have good data to support their safety in pregnancy. It's important to balance a mother's risk of a flare against the theoretical risk of increased birth defects in the fetus. If your disease has been difficult to treat and it's now in remission with these medications, then we recommend that you continue to manage your IBD with 6-MP or azathioprine throughout your pregnancy.

If you really want to be off these medications during pregnancy, you should stop their use at least three months before trying to conceive. It takes a while for the drugs to completely leave your system. If you're taking one of these medications and think that you might be pregnant, do a pregnancy test immediately. The first six to eight weeks of pregnancy are when the fetal organs develop, and if you're already that far along in the pregnancy, stopping use of the medication just puts your disease at risk and doesn't prevent fetal exposure. Whether to continue or stop these medications during pregnancy is an individual decision, and a one-size-fits-all approach is not appropriate here.

For a pregnant woman with severe ulcerative colitis that isn't responding to intravenous steroids, the medications cyclosporine and infliximab can be safer than surgery. Fortunately, the need to use these drugs is rare. A pregnant woman with an ulcerative colitis flare often requires management by a gastroenterologist, an obstetrician and sometimes a surgeon.

The safety of biologic medications is an active area of research. Remicade and infliximab biosimilars have been used the most, with no apparent increased risk to the fetus or the mother. Studies have found that Remicade does cross the placenta, but it's metabolized over time and doesn't appear to affect an infant's immune system. For women on Remicade, it's generally recommended that the dose not be increased as a mother's weight increases during pregnancy. Other IBD medications aren't weight-based for dosing, so the same doses can be continued. There isn't as much data for the newer biologics, but it's logical to assume that they wouldn't increase the rate of birth defects.

Endoscopy procedures during pregnancy

There's generally no need for routine procedures during pregnancy, but if one is required to assess disease activity or obtain tissue samples, then a flexible sigmoidoscopy is usually adequate. Rarely is a full colonoscopy necessary. Flexible sigmoidoscopies can be performed with a tap water enema prep and little or no sedation. There's no evidence to suggest that undergoing a flexible sigmoidoscopy increases the risk for premature rupture of membranes, premature contractions or other problems with pregnancy.

Delivery

In general, women with IBD can have a vaginal delivery unless, for other reasons, a C-section is recommended. If you have active perianal disease at delivery, having a C-section avoids worsening the condition due to the trauma of the birthing process.

If you have a J pouch, a vaginal delivery won't harm the pouch. However, some surgeons recommend that you have a C-section anyway to help retain proper anal sphincter function. A vaginal delivery can compromise the function of the anal sphincter, with or without a pouch. This may happen immediately from the trauma of the pushing during delivery, or it may happen later, even decades later, similar to the aging process that causes muscles in the pelvic floor to sag, increasing the risk of urinary and fecal incontinence.

Breastfeeding

This is a personal decision and shouldn't be forced on you. You must decide whether you want to nurse your baby and then factor in your medications, because having to stop taking them may worsen your condition.

- Breastfeeding *isn't* recommended if you're on antibiotics.
- Breastfeeding *isn't* allowed if you're taking cyclosporine.

- Breastfeeding *isn't* allowed if you're taking a small molecule medication.
- Breastfeeding *is* allowed if you're taking steroids.
- Breastfeeding *is* allowed if you're taking a 5-ASA drug.
- Breastfeeding *is* allowed if you're on azathioprine or 6-MP.
- Breastfeeding *is* allowed if you're taking a biologic.

A final note for nursing mothers: Use of the herbal supplement fenugreek to try to enhance milk production isn't recommended. Some lactation consultants recommend it, but it can cause rectal bleeding, which is obviously not good if you have Crohn's disease or ulcerative colitis.

13

Growing up with IBD

Tyler had always been the "runt" of the class. He never complained of anything, but there were days when he just couldn't keep up with the other kids on the playground. When he reached sixth grade, his parents felt that there might be something wrong. They took him to a pediatrician, who found that Tyler was anemic and iron deficient. Tyler said he'd never seen blood in his stools, and he didn't complain of pain. However, he had learned to stay away from fried foods because they made him feel bad. A CT scan revealed that a portion of his small intestine was inflamed, and a colonoscopy with biopsies revealed that he had Crohn's disease. Tyler began taking methotrexate, folic acid, a biologic and a multivitamin with iron. He started to gain weight and had much more energy.

Perhaps you've just learned that your child has IBD. You may be relieved to finally know what's been causing your child's symptoms but saddened because you've now entered an unknown world.

It's difficult to stay calm and focus on managing the problem when you're wondering if there was something that you could have done to prevent your child's disease. Don't spend your energy

WHAT CAUSED YOUR CHILD'S IBD?

As mentioned in Chapter 1, it's not known why someone develops IBD; however, the matter is being actively studied. There seems to be a genetic component, although no particular gene or combination of genes has been definitively identified as the cause. Here are some facts:

- Just 30% of individuals diagnosed have a family history of IBD.
- The chance of passing IBD to a child is low, roughly 3% to 7%.
- If both parents have IBD, the chance of their child developing IBD increases to almost 50%.

Some people blame the development of Crohn's disease on childhood vaccinations, similar to the thinking that vaccines increase the risk of autism. But the research is definitive: Vaccinations don't cause IBD!

on feeling guilty. While research has provided information on how to manage IBD, little is known about how to prevent the disease. Autoimmune diseases like IBD seem to have both a genetic component and an environmental trigger, and the trigger or combination of triggers may be unique to each individual.

Certainly, it's natural to have questions, concerns and even fears. Other parents and children are looking for answers and support just like you are. You might be surprised to learn that about a quarter of the people in the United States who have IBD are younger than age 18. Children and teens experience the same symptoms and mostly the same issues with IBD as do adults, but there are key differences.

The most common age at diagnosis is 12 and a half years, but children as young as age 3 can develop IBD. In the preschool years, ulcerative colitis is as common as Crohn's disease. However, this shifts with age; more school-age children develop Crohn's disease than ulcerative colitis by approximately 3 to 1.

Developing a chronic disease at age 12 is a big deal. Most children at this age are very self-conscious about their changing bodies and challenged by the rising hormone tides that accompany the teen years. They're more awkward and off balance physically and emotionally than they've ever been in their lives. As they move from elementary school to middle or high school, they feel the desire to not stand out as different from everyone else. What a time to add a chronic disease with symptoms that are difficult to manage and deeply embarrassing.

Fortunately, children and teens are strong and capable. Your bewildered child will develop resiliency. Some even find humor in the situation. These are valuable traits to have when dealing with a chronic disease that can't be cured and must be managed for life. Don't be afraid to let your child take some responsibility — learning when to take medications and what to eat. But know that children with a chronic illness, including IBD, need support and encouragement and, most of all, your hugs when all the right choices don't keep the illness in remission. No one can manage IBD perfectly, and letting go of perfectionism might be a step in the right direction. Your role as parents? Cheerleaders!

Another step in the right direction is to acknowledge both your own and your child's feelings as they arise. Give the feelings a place to sit at your table and keep the conversation going. Acknowledge the new facts of life for your household and figure out the best way to live with them. A chronic illness affects everyone in the family. Work together to define the new normal in your lives.

GROWTH AND DEVELOPMENT

Growing and developing is the primary activity of childhood. This requires a lot of energy, all fueled by food. So it's especially tough to deal with a gastrointestinal illness when you're young. It is easier to notice when children are having difficulty absorbing nutrients because children grow and change so quickly compared to adults. Failure to grow is often the first symptom doctors see, even before gastrointestinal symptoms present

themselves. It's not normal for children to lose weight, but it's typical in children with IBD.

Crohn's disease seems to pose a bigger challenge to growth than does ulcerative colitis. About a third of children are dealing with failure to grow when they're diagnosed with Crohn's disease, whereas only about 10% of children diagnosed with ulcerative colitis are classified this way. The most common cause of growth failure is malnutrition due to absorbing too few calories. This points to issues with the small intestine. A child with a diagnosis of ulcerative colitis experiencing growth failure needs to be thoroughly examined for possible involvement of the small intestine in his or her disease.

Malnutrition and failure to grow can lead to delayed puberty. This can be reversed if the growth plates in the bones haven't fused shut, as was the case with Tyler. Fusing of the plates usually happens around age 15, and Tyler had just turned 12 at diagnosis. Treating Tyler's underlying inflammation and supplementing his diet with depleted nutrients helped greatly to bring on growth spurts and ensure that Tyler matured properly. His parents worked hard to balance his treatment with keeping his routine as normal as possible, so that the emphasis was on Tyler and his ability to get past this, not on his IBD.

DIFFERENCES IN CHILDREN AND TEENS

The nature of IBD is different in children and adults. In children, there's often more inflammation in the upper parts of the digestive tract, meaning the jejunum, stomach and esophagus. This translates into potentially different symptoms than in adults. Inflammation of this part of the small intestine often leads to more vague abdominal pain, stomach inflammation, nausea and vomiting and trouble swallowing.

If your child is diagnosed with either ulcerative colitis or Crohn's disease, it's important for a gastroenterologist to investigate the entire gastrointestinal tract for evidence of disease in more unusual places.

Crohn's disease in children and teens historically tends to be more aggressive and involve more surgeries because it doesn't respond as well to medication as it does in adults, which we call medically refractory disease.

In other words, medicines used to treat adults don't seem to work for children. One way to identify aggressive IBD — disease that may require stronger treatment earlier in the disease course — is blood tests that look for certain proteins (markers). We know of four different markers associated with the presence of IBD.

Research shows that children with more markers and markers at higher concentrations tend to have more aggressive disease than children who have no markers or markers at low concentrations. Children with extensive or highly inflamed IBD need to be treated aggressively, using immunomodulator and

biologic medications. Children who are started on steroids could become dependent on these drugs and, if they need to take them for a long time to calm their disease, fail to grow.

Another major concern is the increased risk of colorectal cancer in people who have IBD for a long time (see Chapter 8). That's why among adults who develop IBD as children, doctors need to be vigilant in screening them for cancer earlier than usual. Specifically, developing ulcerative colitis before age 15 is a known risk factor for the development of colon cancer well before age 50. Your child needs periodic screening colonoscopies — at diagnosis and after eight years, which is the same schedule as for adults with IBD.

TREATING IBD IN CHILDREN AND TEENS

The goals of IBD treatment are essentially the same for children and teens as for adults: Control active inflammation and prevent complications. The first line of therapy for young people with mild to moderate ulcerative colitis, and some children and teens with Crohn's disease, is a 5-ASA medication. Children who have mild Crohn's disease of the small bowel or colon can be treated with budesonide. However, most children with Crohn's disease need alternative medications to control the disease, such as immunomodulators and biologic agents.

Immunomodulators such as 6-mercaptopurine, azathioprine and methotrexate can be effective therapies in children.

Tiffany was diagnosed with ulcerative colitis at age 7. From the beginning, her parents said she refused to take her medications and was difficult. Tiffany didn't think there was anything wrong with her. She hid her medicines under the bed instead of taking them. She minimized her symptoms, but her parents said that she would spend hours in the bathroom in the morning before school and then after school. Tiffany refused to take lunch to school with her, telling her parents that she wasn't hungry during the day. When she entered high school, her parents were concerned that she'd develop an eating disorder and thought that she should be seen by a gastroenterologist who cares for adults.

Tiffany told the gastroenterologist that the medications prescribed to her tasted "icky" and had to be taken too many times a day. She felt alone because she was an only child and thought her parents focused way too much on her disease. She had never met anyone else with ulcerative colitis. The gastroenterologist changed her medications to take just twice daily and suggested she spend a week at a camp sponsored by the Crohn's & Colitis Foundation to meet other kids with ulcerative colitis. For Tiffany, that week was a life-changing, heartening experience. She went to camp every summer after that and later became a camp counselor, which piqued her interest in pursuing a medical career to help kids with chronic illness.

They're used so that steroids can be avoided, or a child can be weaned off steroids. In the past, immunomodulators were the next step if 5-ASA medications didn't work or stopped working. Today, in both children and adults, use of immunomodulators alone is less common because of the development of more effective medications.

Infections are more common in children taking immunomodulators. Unfortunately, schools are where infections tend to be shared quite readily. Watch your child for indications of a developing infection, and encourage handwashing and other sanitary behaviors to help protect against infections.

Your child should receive an annual flu shot. However, children on immunomodulators shouldn't receive any live vaccines, such as the intranasal influenza or chickenpox vaccine. This is because a live vaccine is designed to purposely give the patient a little dose of the disease so that the body can develop a defense against it. Among children and adults who are immunosuppressed, introducing an infection often will lead to a worse infection and not necessarily immunity down the line.

The medication infliximab (Remicade) is used to treat severe Crohn's disease in children because it has very high response rates and avoids the use of steroids. In addition, rates of growth in young patients are much higher if they take infliximab rather than steroids. Studies are taking place involving other biologics, adalimumab (Humira), vedolizumab (Entyvio) and ustekinumab (Stelara). Deciding to use a biologic is a big step because it needs to be taken consistently. Chapter 6 explains why this is so.

In addition to prescribing medications to control inflammation, doctors will pay close attention to your child's growth. If your child isn't growing as expected, nutritional supplementation becomes an important part of the treatment. This may include high-protein or high-calorie supplements, including protein shakes, nutrition drinks and even tube feeding at night for extra calories. Steroids, which can significantly hamper a child's growth, shouldn't be used. If steroids are needed to treat flares, they're for short-term use only — no more than a few weeks.

If your child needs surgery, the procedures are similar to those for adults. Specialized pediatric surgeons operate on children and usually care for them until age 18. If your daughter needs to have her colon removed because of ulcerative colitis, have a discussion with her and her doctors about safeguarding her future fertility. As discussed in Chapter 12, the J-pouch procedure is associated with decreased fertility in about 50% of women. Although this may not be a concern when your daughter is 10 years old, it could be when she is older.

Remember that what and how your child eats can determine how well she or he copes with IBD. Meeting with a nutritionist skilled in IBD can help you better understand your child's nutritional needs and create meal plans designed to meet those needs. For a week or so in advance of your visit, keep a daily food diary to gather information that will be most useful to the nutritionist, who will want to know what kind of foods you serve at home and your child's personal likes and dislikes.

MONITORING IBD IN CHILDREN AND TEENS

Laboratory testing, endoscopy and X-rays are the cornerstones for diagnosis and assessment of IBD. With children and teens, some important factors need to be taken into consideration. Computerized tomography (CT) scans should be used only when necessary to minimize exposure to radiation. More often, magnetic resonance imaging (MRI), which doesn't involve ionizing radiation, is used, along with other forms of noninvasive testing.

Stool tests that look for certain proteins — such as lactoferrin and calprotectin — can reveal active inflammation. The tests can help avoid the need for endoscopy, which requires general anesthesia for young patients, not just conscious sedation as with adults. General anesthesia is used until around age 15, but this depends a lot on the gastroenterologist, the practice patterns in that part of the country and parental and patient preferences.

Even if your child can't express it, he or she may fear an invasive procedure, and the prep for a colonoscopy isn't fun either. Video capsule endoscopy — swallowing a pill containing a camera — may be used in children and adolescents.

Your child may need X-rays to assess bone growth. Bone density scans performed in adults may not be accurate in children. A plain X-ray of the arm can provide information about a child's growth potential when compared to typical progress at his or her chronological age.

Blood protein tests can be helpful to monitor your child's condition. Children with particularly aggressive disease have multiple markers, several of which are currently being studied, and they appear in very high concentrations. It would make sense, then, to use these markers to predict the progress of the disease. The markers appear to be most helpful in children with disease in their small intestine. The more markers present, and the higher their concentration, the more aggressive initial treatment should be.

But it's important to put these markers into the context of the overall clinical picture. The health care team must consider, for example, what the child eats, whether there's secondhand smoke in the home, and how well the child gets along with other family members. These are all factors that have an impact on disease severity: Food may make gastrointestinal symptoms worse, secondhand smoke makes Crohn's disease worse and a stressful family life will affect the course of the disease.

STAYING ON MEDICATION

It might not seem like a difficult task to have your child take medication every day. But all sorts of things can interfere with this: how sick your child is, the level of family support, the involvement of the health care team and so on. It's tempting to stop the medication when IBD is in remission. Your child feels better, and medication can create undesirable side effects.

There are other factors that can make a child resist medication. Perhaps your child is being teased about being sick or being different. Maybe your family is embarrassed by your child's condition and wants to hide it. Maybe the cost of medication is causing your family financial difficulty. Children are sensitive to such issues. All sorts of factors influence how well a patient follows a doctor's advice.

One way to deal with this is to be a good role model. Children will emulate the attitudes and health behaviors of the adults who surround them. Everyone has personal challenges to face; perhaps you can show your child a consistent, healthy approach to something that's a chronic issue for you, like quitting smoking, losing weight or getting more exercise each day.

Ask your child's doctor if it's possible to minimize the pill count or simplify the timing of doses so that medication doesn't need to be taken at school. If your child is permitted to carry personal medication at school, maybe the medication can be kept in a nondescript container. At home, perhaps you can build a routine for pill taking that has everyone taking something, even a multivitamin, so your child with IBD doesn't feel different from everyone else. If your child has a hard time swallowing pills or capsules, perhaps taking them with food will help.

A great resource for children and adolescents who are newly diagnosed with IBD comes from the Crohn's & Colitis Foundation. It's called "Pete Learns All About Crohn's and Colitis" and can be downloaded from the foundation's website (see page 183).

FITTING IN WITH IBD

Children with IBD want so much to fit in and not be different from their peers. The pressure of keeping their disease a secret can be difficult, but children with IBD aren't likely to tell other children about their illness for fear that they'll be teased or rejected. A sympathetic teacher might include a lesson on IBD to raise awareness of the disease with other students without singling out your child. But doing so could lead to bathroom humor jokes and embarrass your child further.

It takes a balanced, calm approach to teach children about this disease. Your child's teachers should be able to help you evaluate the maturity and kindness of your child's classmates and predict how they'll handle the information. Certainly, your child should think about adding best friends to his or her support team. The Crohn's & Colitis Foundation offers educational booklets for teachers that can be downloaded from the foundation's website (see page 183).

What can't be hidden are the aesthetic and emotional side effects of certain medications, steroids in particular. Weight gain — a "moon" face — and irritability are typical with chronic steroid use and can significantly affect how well your child gets along with family and friends at home and at school. Fortunately, other medications don't affect a child's appearance or emotional stability.

Pay attention to your child's state of mind. As with adults, depression and anxiety can develop in children with IBD. Their disease may present them with many challenges that seem overwhelming. Missing a lot of school because of flares and hospitalization can impact your child's school performance and relationships with classmates. Absence from school may draw attention and curiosity from the other children. Does your child get special treatment from teachers? Other children can resent this if they don't understand what's going on. It can be difficult for someone who doesn't have the disease to fully understand what it requires.

Visiting a counselor as a family may provide a supportive place to identify and talk through issues on which a family may be holding back. A psychosocial evaluation for your child and your family can be an important part of the overall management of your child's disease. Medical centers that treat children and teens with IBD often include visits to a social worker or counselor along with visits to doctors. This is because IBD affects more than the body — it also affects the mind and emotions. Such visits are a vital part of overall care.

You might consider having your child join a peer support group to better understand how to live with IBD and to find the motivation to do all that's required. Support groups and camps for children with IBD can play a very important role in helping children and family members cope with IBD. Teens, especially, may acquire new negotiation skills and feel empowered to take better care of themselves.

Most importantly, remember that this is your child's body and your child's disease. Even if your child is only 8 years old, he or she is capable of managing some aspects of the disease. Believe that your child has what it takes to manage IBD, and communicate this to your child and the rest of your family.

Children are quite resilient, especially when they're treated with respect and dignity. The maturity and insight of young patients — some of whom have been dealing with this disease since early childhood — often is humbling.

There are some issues that are common areas of concern among parents raising a child with IBD. Perhaps you find yourself grappling with some of the following situations.

Who gets to know

Talking to other people about your child's disease may not seem like a big issue, but there's actually much to consider before relaying information to others. There are many reasons why parents want to discuss a child's new diagnosis with others. First, most parents are understandably feeling very emotional and have countless questions about the illness. Health is a very emotional issue, and parents often want to talk to others about their child's IBD because they're upset and talking is a common way to react to such problems.

Parents can begin their research by asking other parents of children with IBD for names of physicians and hospitals to help learn more about what may be in store for their child and their family. Another resource is the Crohn's & Colitis Foundation (see page 183), which has multiple education programs available, including programs for children and adolescents newly diagnosed with IBD.

Sometimes, parents are so caught up in their own emotions and concerns that they don't think about the fact that they're discussing their children's private body parts and bathroom habits. Their children may not respond favorably to knowing that others are finding out about their disease. An effective approach is to discuss with your child who should know, then respect their boundaries. Imagine if they went to school and shared with their friends that Mom spent hours in the bathroom with bloody diarrhea!

Asking how your child is feeling

One goal of parenting a child with IBD involves building a healthy identity for your child. For example, your 10th-grade son is a member of the debate team, an editor of the student newspaper, an honor roll student and a member of the tennis team. This gives him the opportunity to enjoy a healthy, robust identity as a successful student.

Now let's assume your son, this same boy, develops Crohn's disease and spends time being hospitalized, receiving infusions, and having to discuss his disease with his teachers. Let's also assume that each day, his caring family and support team want to know how he's feeling. Your son would prefer to focus on the positive, enjoyable parts of his life — being on the debate team, editing the newspaper, and so on. But because he is constantly being asked how he is feeling, he's forced to think about the painful, negative parts.

If two grandparents each ask once a day how he's feeling, and each parent asks twice, and two teachers ask once, and the tennis coach asks once, and his older sister asks once, and then mom asks him

if he took his medication before he went to bed, this teen is being redirected to think about his illness many more times than necessary. This is how families and friends run the risk of transforming this boy's identity from an active 10th grader to a sick child.

Despite your great intentions, this can hinder your child's healthy development. Consider establishing limits of inquiry with your child in which only one parent asks once a day how your son or daughter is feeling. You can also ask friends and family to limit their questions. In exchange for setting such boundaries, your child has to agree to be totally honest about how he or she feels or symptoms that he or she may be experiencing.

Sometimes, children are so afraid of the repercussions of their symptoms, including needing to take more medication or having more doctor visits, that they don't share all the information. Make sure your child knows that it's OK to raise the issue on his or her own at any time. Open dialogue is very important.

Medication compliance

Parents will often say that they're so grateful that their children take their medications regularly and that medication compliance isn't an issue. Meanwhile, in a separate session next door, a child is telling facilitators about tossing, flushing or hiding medication or even feeding it to the family dog! It's safe to say that almost all children become noncompliant with their medications at some point during their teenage years. Typically, it's when they're feeling well and naively think that a few weeks off isn't a big deal. Unfortunately, these same teens may end up missing prom or the school play and even having surgery because of noncompliance.

Because the stakes are so high, doctors often encourage parents to actually watch their children take their medication. This needs to be done with great tact and sensitivity. In a nonchalant manner, parents should establish a morning or evening routine (or both, depending on when the child needs to take medication). Perhaps the medication is kept in the kitchen, and your child takes it before breakfast or after dinner when you're nearby.

Some children will respond with comments such as, "You don't trust me!" We encourage parents to explain that it isn't a matter of trust — taking medication for an illness every day is hard for anyone, and you want to show support by being there with them during that difficult part of their day. Throwing in a favorite drink that doesn't exacerbate their symptoms is also helpful in sweetening the whole experience.

How to make swallowing pills easier

Watch children eat, and you'll notice that most of them don't chew their food well. In fact, parents can often be heard saying to younger children, "Take smaller bites and chew!" Softer foods such as macaroni and cheese or vegetable soup get swallowed without much chewing. This is important to remember if your child is struggling to swallow pills.

Difficulty swallowing pills probably means that a child is simply afraid — not just of the pills but of all the changes and experiences that he or she is going through. Let your child know that you understand these changes are scary and that pills can be tough to take, even for grown-ups, and sometimes pills leave a bad aftertaste. But also convey that medication plays a big part in making your child feel well. The more a child can equate pills with feeling better, the more willing he or she may be to take them.

Try not to pressure your child about his or her pills. The more stressed out you are, the more stressed out your child will be and the less successful he or she will be at swallowing them. Show them that it's possible to eat some food, such as applesauce or a small spoonful of macaroni and cheese, without chewing. Spoonfuls of these foods are larger than most IBD pills. Some parents begin by putting a pill inside a tube-shaped noodle and serving it with a plate of macaroni. While the child is eating, distract him or her with conversation. Before you know it, your son or daughter will have consumed mouthfuls of the food and the pill with it.

The most important thing to remember is that the more relaxed and calm you are, the better. Your child will get there. Over time, even children who struggle with pills become pros at taking several large pills at a time.

Guiding children to independence

In adolescence, there's a natural progression of children growing into independent adults. During that time, parents gradually lessen their involvement in the decisions their children make. For example, whereas parents are more likely to be involved in structuring a child's activities when he or she is younger, a teenager will progressively make his or her own decisions regarding whom to spend time with and in what activities to engage. That's a healthy, natural process in which a child grows into an autonomous adult.

When disease is part of the picture, parents often have less ability to let go. They naturally tighten their grip as a child faces new realities and tries to become more independent. This can have a detrimental impact. A child with IBD very often has been traumatized by pain, the need for medical procedures and hospitalization, and may already may be somewhat dependent on you. Trying to stifle the natural desire for independence that comes with adolescence may cause your son or daughter to regress into an even more dependent state.

One way that parents can assist their child in the journey to greater independence is to allow him or her to "take ownership" of the IBD. Depending on your child's age and maturity level, begin by letting him or her speak at doctor visits. This may sound obvious, but many parents answer basic questions for their child, including "How are you feeling?" and "How many bowel movements are you having a day?" It's imperative to allow a child to begin to speak for himself or herself.

Even a young child can answer simple questions and very often knows the answers better than his or her parents. Remember, the symptoms are occurring in your child's body! By the later teenage years, a child should be encouraged to fully speak for himself or herself, and parents may stay in the waiting room during appointments.

IBD at school

One of the main challenges of having IBD for children and teens is dealing with the disease at school. For some lucky teens, it's rarely an issue and most bathroom activity occurs early in the morning or after school. But most kids and teens need to figure out how to handle issues such as taking medications at school, getting to the bathroom in time, explaining absences, and taking part in activities when they feel sick and exhausted.

With your child's permission, before the school year starts, meet with your child's teachers and make them aware of the IBD and its symptoms so that they can support your child. For example, teachers will often allow students with IBD to leave class without asking permission so they can use the bathroom whenever necessary, with the understanding that the privilege won't be abused.

If your child's school or teachers aren't cooperative and understanding, you might check into programs such as a Section 504 Plan, which is part of the Americans with Disabilities Act. Each 504 Plan is individualized for a specific student's needs. It outlines the modifications and accommodations necessary for a particular student to perform at the same level as his or her peers.

For a student with IBD, the accommodations might include bathroom access whenever needed, freedom to use staff bathrooms to increase privacy, exemptions from certain physical education activities when the student doesn't feel well, extra time to complete assignments if the student isn't well and allowance for tardiness in the morning, a time when IBD is often more active. A 504 Plan can give a student a sense of comfort knowing that IBD won't hamper his or her ability to succeed in school.

Additional resources

Contact these organizations for more information about inflammatory bowel disease.

American College of Gastroenterology
www.gi.org

American Gastroenterological Association
www.gastro.org

Crohn's & Colitis Foundation
www.crohnscolitisfoundation.org

IBD Support Foundation
www.ibdsf.org

Inflammatory Bowel Disease Center — Mount Sinai
www.myibd.org

Mayo Clinic
www.MayoClinic.org

National Institutes of Health
www.nih.gov

U.S. National Library of Medicine (clinical trials database)
www.clinicaltrials.gov

The J-Pouch Group
www.j-pouch.org

We Care (A support group for women with IBD who are pregnant or planning pregnancy.)
www.wecareinibd.com

United Ostomy Associations of America
www.ostomy.org

Index

A

abscess, 119
aminosalicylates, 63-65, 72
anastomotic ischemia, 120
anastomotic leak, 119
anemia, 157
ankylosing spondylitis, 97
antibiotics, 73-75
antidiarrheals, 82-83
anti-inflammatory medications. *See also*
    medications
    about, 61
    aminosalicylates, 63-65, 72
    steroids, 61-63, 72, 97, 122, 174-175
anxiety, 155-156
arthralgia, 97
ASCA marker, 47
autoimmune hepatitis, 93-94
autoimmune reaction, 15
avascular necrosis (AVN), 97

B

balloon-assisted enteroscopy, 44
barium studies, 42
biologics. *See also* medications
    about, 67-68
    children and teens and, 175
    example case, 71
    newer, 70-71
    older adults and, 72
    Pap tests and, 163-164
    pregnancy and, 168
    risks, 70
    side effects of, 69-70
    summary, 71
    types of, 68-69
    working of, 68
biopsies, 32
biosimilars, 69
bleeding, 39, 45, 114
blood clots, 118-119, 165

blood tests, 29, 41-42, 176
body-affected areas
    bones, 95-97
    eyes, 9-23
    hair, teeth and nails, 97-98
    joints, 97
    kidneys, 94-95
    liver, 93-94
    skin, 98-99
bone density scans, 176
bones and IBD, 95-97
bowel. *See* colon
bowel movements, ulcerative colitis and,
    27-28
bowel obstruction, 119
breastfeeding, 169-170

C

C. difficile **infection,** 42, 73-75, 85
calcium, 128, 137-138
calories, 141
cancer
    cholangiocarcinoma, 105
    colorectal, 100-103
    lymphoma, 66-67, 70, 72, 103-105
    rare tumors, 105-106
Candida, 29
capsule endoscopy, 43-44
carbohydrates, 125, 126
cause of IBD
    environment and, 20-21
    genetics and, 18-19
    immune system and, 19-20
    theories, 18
celiac disease, 139-140
children and teens with IBD
    about, 170-172
    causes, 171
    common diagnosis age, 171
    differences in, 172-173
    example cases, 170, 174

    fitting in and, 177-178
    growth and development and, 172
    guiding to independence, 181
    immunomodulators for, 173-174
    infections and, 174
    inquiries on how feeling and, 179, 181
    malnutrition and, 172
    medication compliance, 179-180
    medications and, 173-174, 175, 176-177
    monitoring, 175-176
    parental issues, 178–182
    school and, 177-178, 181-182
    surgery and, 175
    swallowing pills and, 180
    treating, 173-175
    who gets to know and, 178-179
cholangiocarcinoma, 105
clinical trials, 85-86
codeine, 83
collagenous colitis, 48-49
colon
    about, 14
    fiber and, 132
    illustrated, 15, 27, 38
    images, 31
    layers, 14
    mucosa, 14
    removal, 110-112
colonoscopy
    biopsies, 32, 102-103
    children and teens and, 176
    colon cleansing preparations for, 30, 31
    in colorectal cancer prevention,
        101-102
    Crohn's disease and, 43
    examination, 29-31
    images, 31
    procedure, 32
    sedative medications, 31-32
    ulcerative colitis and, 29-32
colorectal cancer
    about, 100

colorectal cancer continued
    colonoscopies and, 101-102
    dysplasia and, 102-103
    example case, 102
    medications to prevent, 103
    prevention, 101-102
    risk factors, 100-101
colostomy, 121
complementary therapies
    about, 87-88
    categories of, 88
    not proved to work for IBD, 89
    prebiotics, 91
    probiotics, 90-91
    safety and, 88
computerized tomography (CT), 42-43, 44
constipation, ulcerative colitis and, 28
continent ostomy, 122
contraception, 164-165
corticosteroids, 72
COVID-19, 57-58
Crohn's & Colitis Foundation, 6, 18, 54, 174, 177
Crohn's colitis, 39
Crohn's disease. *See also* children and teens with IBD; inflammatory bowel disease (IBD)
    about, 37-38
    as chronic condition, 45
    diagnosis, 40-44
    in esophagus, 40
    example cases, 37, 39, 40
    fistulas, 38-39, 67, 85, 117
    flares, 21, 22, 44-45, 129-130, 145-147
    IBS and, 17
    inflammation and, 37-39
    managing, 44-45
    MAP and, 21
    pain and, 84
    scar tissue, 39
    of the small intestine, 106
    statistics, 15-16

    surgery and, 108
    symptoms, 39-40
    types of, 38-39
    understanding, 37-45
Crohn's disease, surgery for
    about, 108, 109, 115-116
    fistulas and, 117
    hemorrhoids and skin tags and, 117-118
    perforation or abscess repair, 116-117
    reasons for, 116
    resection, 108, 109, 116
Crohn's ileitis, 39
CT enterography (CTE), 42-43

D

dehydration, 28
depression, 21, 23, 155-156
diagnosing Crohn's disease
    about, 40
    imaging and, 42-44
    physical exam and, 41
    questions in, 40
    tests and, 41-42
diagnosing ulcerative colitis
    about, 28
    colonoscopy and, 29-32
    medical history and, 29
    in older adults, 32-34
    tests and, 29
diagnosis, IBD
    confirming, 17-18
    IBD vs. IBS and, 17
    misdiagnosis and, 16-17
    outcomes and, 18
    primary care discussion and, 55
diarrhea, 27-28, 39, 45, 48, 49, 120
diet(s). *See also* foods; nutrition
    about, 143-145
    after flare recovery, 149
    changing, 145
    during flare, 145-147

for IBD, 143-149
low-residue, 150
Mediterranean diet, 127, 143-145
normal, getting back to, 148
Specific Carbohydrate Diet, 143-145
when you start to feel better, 147-148
dual-energy X-ray absorptiometry (DXA or DEXA) scan, 96
dysplasia, 102-103

E

eating disorders and IBD, 22
enteral nutrition, 142-143, 150
environment and IBD, 20-21
enzymes, 150
erythema nodosum, 98
exercising, 157-158
eyes and IBD, 92-93

F

family members, informing of diagnosis, 24
fatigue, 156-157
fats, 125, 126-128, 151
fecal microbiota transfer (FMT), 74-75
fertility, 165-166
fever, 28, 39
fiber
about, 131-132
adding, 134-135
flares and, 129
guidelines, 134
types of, 132
fish oil, 90
fistulas. *See also* Crohn's disease
about, 38-39
defined, 117
medications and, 67, 73
stem cells for, 85
treating, 117

5-ASA (5-aminosalicylic acid), 63-64, 74-77, 87, 94-95, 174
504 Plan, 182
flares
about, 21, 22
causes of, 35
Crohn's disease, 44-45
defined, 35
diet and, 129-130
eating during, 145-147
ulcerative colitis, 35-36
folate, 120-121
folic acid, 142, 167
food allergies, 140
food diary, 131
foods. *See also* nutrition
feeling better, 147-148
fiber, 129, 131-134
during flare, 145-147
flare recovery, 149
getting back to normal, 148-149
gluten and, 139-140
in IBD-modified diets, 129
lactose intolerance and, 135-137
red meat, 130
trigger, 138-139

G

gallstones, 94
gastrointestinal (GI) tract, 13, 14-15, 20
genetics and IBD, 18-19
GI specialty center, 58-59
gluten, 139-140, 150
goals, 54-55, 56
growing up with IBD. *See* children and teens with IBD
gut microbiome, 133, 143

H

hair, teeth, nails and IBD, 97

health care team, 56-59
hemorrhoids, 117-118
hepatitis B, 70
hepatosplenic T-cell lymphoma, 104-105
heredity and IBD, 19
hormone replacement therapy, 163
humoral immunity, 20
hydrocortisone, 74-75
hyperbaric oxygen, 85

I

IBD. *See* inflammatory bowel disease
IBS (irritable bowel syndrome), 17
ileoanal anastomosis, 113
ileostomy, 52, 121
ileum, 20
ileus, 118
imaging, 42-44
immune system and IBD, 19-20
immunomodulators. *See also* medications
    about, 65
    azathioprine, 65–66, 72, 76–77, 94, 168,
        173-174
    characteristics of, 76-77
    cyclosporine, 67, 76-77
    effectiveness and side effects of, 65-66
    methotrexate, 66-67, 76-77, 94, 167,
        173-174
    Pap tests and, 163-164
    6-mercaptopurine, 65-66, 72, 76-77, 94,
        168, 173-174
    tacrolimus, 67, 76-77
indeterminate colitis, 46-47
inflammation
    about, 15
    Crohn's disease and, 37-39
    IBD and, 17
    illustrated, 15
    immune system and, 19
    indeterminate colitis and, 46, 47
    microscopic colitis and, 47-48
    perspective, 127
    TNF and, 20
    ulcerative colitis and, 26, 27, 32
inflammation of the pouch (pouchitis), 114
inflammatory bowel disease (IBD).
        See also Crohn's disease; ulcerative
        colitis
innate immunity, 20
intermediate plan, 51-52
iritis, 92
iron, 142
irritable bowel syndrome (IBS), 17

J

Janus kinase (JAK) inhibitors, 85
jejunostomy, 121
J-pouch procedure, 112-113, 115, 165.
        See also pouches

K

kidneys and IBD, 94-95

L

lactase enzyme, 136, 150
lactose intolerance, 135-137
large intestine. *See* colon
leaks, pouch, 113-114
lifestyle issues, 55
liver and IBD, 93-94
long-term plan, 56
loperamide, 82
lymph system, 20
lymphocytic colitis, 47-48
lymphoma
    about, 103-104
    hepatosplenic T-cell, 104-105
    risk, 66, 67, 70, 72, 104
    symptoms, 105
    types of, 104

M

M. paratuberculosis (MAP), 21
macronutrients, 150
magnetic resonance imaging (MRI), 43
malnutrition, 141-142, 151, 172
MAP (*M. paratuberculosis*), 21
medications. *See also specific types*
    about, 60
    aminosalicylates, 63-65, 72
    antibiotics, 73-75
    antidiarrheals, 82-83
    anti-inflammatory, 61-65
    beginning, 51
    biologics, 67-71, 163-164, 168, 175
    clinical trials, 85-86
    in colorectal cancer prevention, 103
    complementary therapies, 87-91
    future treatments, 84-85
    for IBD inflammation (table), 74-81
    immunomodulators, 65-67, 72, 76-77,
        94, 167-168, 173-174
    older adults and urinary incontinence,
        72
    pain, 83-84
    pregnancy and, 167-168
    in short-term plan, 53
    small molecules, 71-73
    staying on, 86-87
    steroids, 34, 61-63, 72, 97, 122, 174-175
    topical, 72, 74-77
Mediterranean diet, 127, 144-145
men and IBD, 160
menopause, 163
menstruation, 162-163
methylprednisolone, 61, 74-75
microbiome, gut, 133, 143
micronutrients, 151
microscopic colitis, 47-48
minerals, 125, 128
misdiagnosis, 16-17
mucus, rectum, 14-15

N

narcotics, 84
nausea and vomiting, 39, 45, 88-90
NOD2 gene, 18, 19
NUDT15 enzyme test, 66
nutrition. *See also* foods
    carbohydrates and, 125, 126
    challenge of, 124-125
    enteral, 142-143, 150
    fats and, 125, 126-128, 151
    fiber and, 129, 131-134
    glutamine and, 140-141
    guidelines, 150-152
    IBD-required modifications, 129-131
    importance of, 125
    individual needs, 129-131
    malnutrition and, 141-142, 172
    minerals and, 125, 128
    needs, 125-129
    oral nutritional supplements, 135, 138,
        142, 151
    parenteral, 143, 151
    proteins and, 125, 126
    vitamins and, 125, 128
    water, 128-129

O

older adults, 32-34, 72
omega-3 fatty acids, 127, 151
oral nutritional supplements, 135, 138, 142,
    151
osteomalacia, 97
osteoporosis, 95-96

P

pain, 84, 153-154
pain medications, 83-84
p-ANCA protein, 47
Pap tests, 163-164

parenteral nutrition, 143, 151
perforation or abscess repair, 116-117
physical activity, 157-158
polyunsaturated fats, 127
postoperative complications, 118-121. *See also* surgery
pouches. *See also* J-pouch procedure
 about, 113
 benefits and drawbacks, 115
 bleeding and cuffitis, 114
 inflammation of, 115, 114
 issues with, 113-115
 leakage, 113-114
 obstruction, 114
 pregnancy and, 169
prednisone, 61, 62, 74-75, 167-168
pregnancy
 breastfeeding and, 169
 delivery and, 169
 endoscopy procedures during, 168-169
 fertility and, 165-166
 IBD and, 166-167
 medications during, 167-168
 planning, 166
 "rule-of-thirds" and, 167
preventive health care measures, 57
primary sclerosing cholangitis, 93
probiotics, 90-91, 114, 136
proteins, 125, 126, 130, 141
pyoderma gangrenosum, 67, 98-99

Q

quality-of-life issues, 55, 113

R

rectal exam, 41
rectum, 14-15, 26-29, 165
resection, 108, 109, 116
residue, 132, 151

S

sacroiliitis, 97
scar tissue, 115
school, children and teens with IBD at, 177-178, 181-182
self-awareness tools, 54
self-management
 about, 50
 intermediate plan, 51-52
 long-term plan, 56
 plans, 50, 51-56
 preventive health care measures and, 57
 short-term plan, 52-55
SER-287, 85
sexuality, 160-162
SHINGRIX shingles vaccine, 73
short bowel syndrome, 121
short-chain fatty acids (SCFAs), 133, 151
short-term plan, 52-55. *See also* self-management
skin and IBD, 98-99
skin tags, 117-118
sleep, 156
small intestine
 about, 14
 attaching to rectum, 165
 Crohn's disease and, 38, 39, 40, 43
 illustrated, 38
 imaging, 43
 measuring length of, 121
small molecules, 71-73
Specific Carbohydrate Diet, 143-145
stem cells, 85
steroids, 34, 61-63, 72, 97, 122, 174, 175
stomas, 121-123
stool tests, 29, 42, 73, 175
stress, 154-155
stricturoplasty, 108-110
surgery. *See also specific surgical procedures*
 about, 107

children and teens and, 175
for Crohn's disease, 115-118
fears, discussing, 55
postoperative complications and, 118-121
steroids and, 122
stomas and, 121-123
summary, 123
terminology, 111
transplant, 110
types of, 108-110
for ulcerative colitis, 110-115
symptom diary, 54
symptoms
    Crohn's disease, 39-40
    general IBD, 12
    ulcerative colitis, 27-28, 33, 34-35

T

tenesmus, 27-28
tests, 29, 41-42. *See also specific tests*
TMPT enzyme test, 66
TNF (tumor necrosis factor), 20
tobacco use, 157
topical medications, 72, 74-77
total parenteral nutrition (TPN), 94, 121
transplant surgery, 110
travel, 158
trigger foods, 138-139
tumor necrosis factor (TNF), 20, 68, 70

U

ulcerative colitis. *See also* children and teens with IBD; inflammatory bowel disease (IBD)
    about, 26-27
    as chronic condition, 36
    diagnosing, 28–34
    flares, 35-36
    IBS and, 17

inflammation and, 26, 27, 32
managing, 34-36
misdiagnosis, 17
"morning rush hour," 28
pain and, 84
statistics, 15-16
symptoms, 27-28, 33, 34-35
treatment determination, 34
treatment factors, 34
understanding, 26-36
ulcerative colitis, surgery for
    about, 110-112
    colon removal, 112-113
    pouches and, 113-115
unsaturated and trans fats, 126-127, 130
uveitis, 92

V

vaccines, 57-58
vitamin B-12, 120
vitamin D, 138, 142
vitamins, 125, 127, 128, 138, 142

W

water, 128-129, 152
weight loss, 39, 48, 55
whey protein isolate, 136-137
women and IBD
    contraception, 164-165
    example case, 162
    menopause, 163
    menstruation, 162-163
    Pap tests, 163-164
    sexuality and, 161-162
workplace, 24-25, 158-159
wound infection, 119

Z

zinc, 142

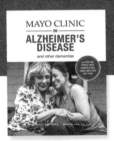
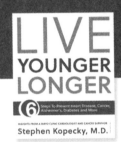
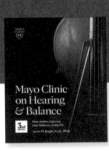
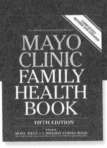
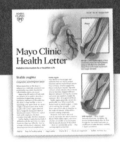